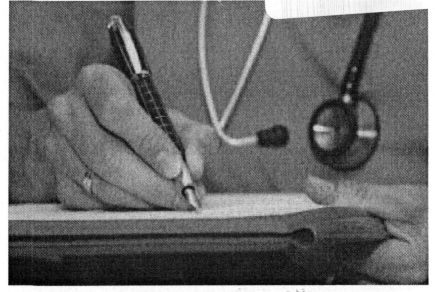

The What, Why and How of Getting into Medical School

The definitive guide by current medical students for future medical students

**Christopher Graham, Dayo Kashimawo,
Michael Thurm, Rajiv Sethi
Edited by Mr Gopal Mahadev
and Matt Green**

BPP
UNIVERSITY
SCHOOL OF HEALTH

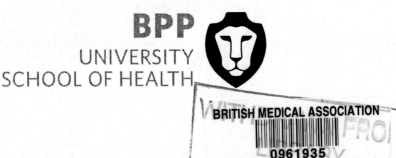

First edition January 2016

ISBN 9781 4727 3897 4
eISBN 9781 4727 3937 7
eISBN 9781 4727 3941 4

British Library Cataloguing-in-Publication Data
A catalogue record for this book is available from
the British Library

Published by
BPP Learning Media Ltd
BPP House, Aldine Place
London W12 8AA

www.bpp.com/health

Printed in the United Kingdom by RICOH UK
Limited

Unit 2
Wells Place
Merstham
RH1 3LG

Your learning materials, published by BPP
Learning Media Ltd, are printed on paper
sourced from sustainable, managed forests.

The views expressed in this book are those of BPP
Learning Media and not those of UCAS or the
NHS. BPP Learning Media are in no way associated
with or endorsed by the UCAS or the NHS.

The contents of this book are intended as a guide
and not professional advice. Although every effort
has been made to ensure that the contents of
this book are correct at the time of going to
press, BPP Learning Media, the Editor and the
Author make no warranty that the information
in this book is accurate or complete and accept
no liability for any loss or damage suffered by
any person acting or refraining from acting as
a result of the material in this book.

Every effort has been made to contact the
copyright holders of any material reproduced
within this publication. If any have been
inadvertently overlooked, BPP Learning Media
will be pleased to make the appropriate credits
in any subsequent reprints or editions.

A note about copyright

Dear Customer

What does the little © mean and
why does it matter?

Your market-leading BPP books,
course materials and e-learning
materials do not write and update
themselves. People write them on
their own behalf or as employees of
an organisation that invests in this
activity. Copyright law protects their
livelihoods. It does so by creating
rights over the use of the content.

Breach of copyright is a form of theft
– as well as being a criminal offence
in some jurisdictions, it is potentially
a serious beach of professional ethics.

With current technology, things
might seem a bit hazy but, basically,
without the express permission of
BPP Learning Media:

- Photocopying our materials is a
  breach of copyright
- Scanning, ripcasting or conversion
  of our digital materials into
  different file formats, uploading
  them to facebook or e-mailing
  them to your friends is a breach
  of copyright

You can, of course, sell your
books, in the form in which you
have bought them – once you
have finished with them. (Is this
fair to your fellow students? We
update for a reason.)   But the
e-products are sold on a single
user license basis: we do not supply
'unlock' codes to people who have
bought them secondhand.

And what about outside the UK?
BPP Learning Media strives to make
our materials available at prices
students can afford by local printing
arrangements, pricing policies and
partnerships which are clearly listed
on our website. A tiny minority ignore
this and indulge in criminal activity by
illegally photocopying our material
or supporting organisations that do.
If they act illegally and unethically in
one area, can you really trust them?

BPP
UNIVERSITY
SCHOOL OF HEALTH

Contents

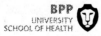

Contents

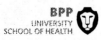

Contents

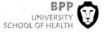

About the publisher

BPP Learning Media is dedicated to supporting aspiring professionals with top quality learning material. BPP Learning Media's commitment to success is shown by our record of quality, innovation and market leadership in paper-based and e-learning materials. BPP Learning Media's study materials are written by professionally qualified specialists who know from personal experience the importance of top quality materials for success.

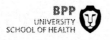

Disclaimer

The answers provided in this book are based on the views of the authors at the time of their applications, to give you an indication of the standard required.

Do not 'lift' answers from this book, as your responses have to be based on truth and your own experiences (and the information may no longer be current or relevant).

Foreword

There is a perception that getting into medical school is like trying to gain entry into an exclusive club. Yes, academic aptitude is important but it is also a matter of who you know and whether you have the right answers to what seem to be a set of closely guarded questions.

Fortunately things are changing, with medical schools tasked by the Medical Schools Council to widen participation to medicine and diversify the people working in the profession. There are now more female than male doctors, a growing number of students from BME backgrounds and more students from abroad choosing to study in the UK. But despite these steps to make medicine more inclusive, there's more work to do, as a mystique still exists around how you actually get a place at medical school.

One of the most challenging aspects of the application process is how to prepare for your interview – and this is a key focus in this book. Up until this point the application process is mostly a science: if you get the right grades, do well in your entrance exams and hone your personal statement, you have a pretty good chance of being invited for an interview.

The challenge that most applicants face is that they have not had many interviews before, let alone one quite like a medical school interview. It's a unique experience: not only are you applying to study on a course at a university, but you are also applying for a profession, that has academic and emotional demands, as well as a set of professional values you will need to uphold for years to come. And then there's the type of interview. Is it a formal panel interview or is it a multiple mini interview? Getting your head around what interviewers are looking for, the format, how to sell yourself, how to address your weaknesses, the complex web of the NHS, can cause applicants to have sleepless nights.

What makes this book stand out as essential preparation for any applicant is that it is written by four medical students who have recently gone through the application process and are all studying at different medical schools. Between them they have experienced many different interview styles. They are not only blessed with

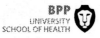

knowing the type of questions medical schools ask applicants but are also mindful of the common concerns applicants have prior to an interview.

Each applicant's journey and reasons for applying to medical school will be unique and it is important to remember this will be your biggest strength at interview stage. (I urge you to read each of the authors' stories of how they got into medical school at the beginning of this book.) Medical school interviews are not meant to be easy and there's no magic formula to getting into medical school, but this book will equip you with the tools and techniques to give yourself the best chance. And now, thanks to the authors, being successful in your medical school application is an open book.

Matthew Billingsley, Editor of The Student BMJ

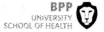

Acknowledgements

The authors would like to express their gratitude to all of the people that helped to make this book a reality; to all those who provided support, offered comments, and assisted with proofreading and editing.

We want to acknowledge and thank the following for their contributions and support:

BPP for enabling us to publish this book;

Matthew Billingsley for supporting the book and writing the foreword;

Vinay Mandagere for proofreading and making suggestions;

Geraldine Jeffers for her time, patience and suggestions;

Dipak Kanabar, for his comments on multiple mini interviews;

Kelvin Chu and Ibrahim Alkurd for offering comments and suggestions;

Altrincham Grammar School for Boys and its staff for their support with our medical school applications;

Gopal Mahadev, for inspiring and supporting Michael, Dayo and Christopher as they successfully applied to medical school;

Last but not least, we would like to thank our families for their unwavering support.

Please note: Any errors or omissions lie with the authors alone.

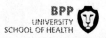

About the authors

Christopher Graham – University of Edinburgh

I first applied to study Medicine in October 2010. I undertook numerous placements to ensure Medicine was what I really wanted to do: dialysis in Spain, general practice, volunteering in a care home, with St John Ambulance, in a hospice and some other voluntary work with children and those in need. I worked hard to achieve 10 A*s and 2 As at GCSE.

I travelled extensively and was active in my school and local community. My peers appointed me as Head Boy. My Personal Statement was therefore quite strong (but improved considerably the next year, in terms of readability and what I had done).

After attending numerous Open Days I opted for: Bristol, Newcastle, Nottingham and Oxford. I had interviews at Bristol and Nottingham, where I underperformed. Although I had practised I felt unsure of myself and lacked confidence. I was pretty gutted (!) to get four rejections. I knew that Medicine was what I wanted to do, so I decided a gap year would be best. I was determined to reapply after strengthening my application.

After achieving strong grades in Maths, Chemistry, Biology and Spanish, I spent the summer working and volunteering for various charities. I got a job as a barman (a great place to work on communication and interpersonal skills). I also worked as a 'relief' caretaker, an invigilator and a cleaner – to raise funds for my studies. More importantly, I shadowed a breast cancer surgeon, who also spent time improving my interview technique and offering advice on my Personal Statement.

I applied to Dundee, Edinburgh, Manchester and Newcastle. I had interviews at Dundee (MMI), Manchester (group interview) and Newcastle (traditional interview). I got offers from Edinburgh (no interview, so strong Personal Statement and high UKCAT score essential) and Manchester.

I opted for Edinburgh because I loved the city and the course sounded well-structured and had a nice balance of problem-based learning and traditional teaching. Furthermore, the students were knowledgeable, confident and down-to-earth!

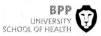

I am very happy and proud to be at Edinburgh. There is a lot to learn, but it's manageable with the right attitude.

I hope this book helps you to achieve your dream.

Dayo Kashimawo – University of Newcastle

I first applied to study Medicine in October 2010. I researched entry requirements and visited the universities I was interested in to see whether I could see myself spending five years there (very important!). I chose Birmingham, Bristol, Keele and Leeds. I achieved good GCSEs of 8 A*s and 3 As which I knew would help with my application to Leeds and especially Birmingham.

Prior to applying, I had volunteered in a nursing home every week for a year. I had also completed a week's work experience in a pharmacy and on a paediatric ward. Unfortunately I didn't receive any interview offers because my Personal Statement wasn't strong enough. It was disappointing, but I was passionate about doing Medicine so I decided to take a year out and apply again. I achieved 3 As at A Level so I had the grades I needed.

During my gap year, I undertook three weeks of work experience shadowing a breast surgeon. I also took the opportunity to improve my Personal Statement and interview techniques to make sure I got my place at Medical School. For the majority of my gap year I worked in the retail sector to earn money for university.

On my second time of applying after extensive research again, I chose Birmingham, Liverpool, Manchester and Newcastle. This time I was more successful and received interview offers from Birmingham, Manchester and Newcastle. Once I received these interviews, I did more interview practice to make sure I was ready. The interviews were daunting but I managed to get offers from Manchester and Newcastle. I chose to go to Newcastle as I preferred an integrated approach to learning, I loved the city, and I also wanted to move away from Manchester.

I am currently starting my clinical years of Medical School and although it can be hard, I am enjoying it thoroughly. I hope this book helps you with your application. If you are passionate about doing Medicine, don't let any hurdles get in your way.

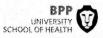

Mike Thurm – University of Manchester

I first applied to study Medicine in October 2010. Prior to my application, I volunteered on a weekly basis at a residential home, as well as completing two work shadowing placements in hospitals to ensure that embarking on a career in Medicine was right for me. I had worked part time in a pharmacy for over a year, completed my Duke of Edinburgh Gold Award, and was Deputy Head Boy of my school with good GCSE grades achieved. Therefore, with the exception of having been predicted a B grade in A Level Biology, I was in a fairly good position when applying to Medical Schools. The universities I applied to were Bristol, Keele, Sheffield and Southampton as they were the only ones that accepted a B grade at the time, and I got offered an interview at Keele. However, I was ill-prepared for my interview and unfortunately did not get offered a place for 2011 entry.

As I was fully committed to studying Medicine, and had achieved three A grades (in Maths, Chemistry and Biology) I persevered at gaining a place at Medical School. I took a gap year and applied again in October 2011. During my year out of education, I undertook a further placement with a breast cancer surgeon who also helped to improve my interview technique and gave me advice on my Personal Statement. I also got a job as a barman at a local hotel and volunteered at a youth club once a week.

On my second attempt, I applied to Leeds, Manchester, Newcastle and Sheffield as I liked their integrated approaches with a mixture of PBL and lectures, and they placed more emphasis on my high UKCAT score. I had interviews at Manchester, Newcastle and Sheffield that all went better than my one the previous year at Keele, and took up my offer to study Medicine at Manchester.

I am now intercalating at Manchester. The workload can sometimes feel quite hard, with a lot to learn, but with a good balance of work and extra-curricular activities it can be managed.

Best wishes with your application, and I hope this book helps you to be successful!

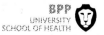

Rajiv Sethi – King's College London

Applying to Medical School can be a stressful time and seem difficult to manage alongside your studies and life. When I applied I remember being overwhelmed by the multitude of resources and specific criteria for various Medical Schools. If only there was a definitive resource to turn to. With this in mind I wanted to work towards creating a 'tell it how it is' guide for prospective medical students.

I organised my first work experience when I was 15. This attachment involved working with the administrators of a nuclear Medicine department. I was limited in what I could observe clinically, however I thoroughly enjoyed the week. I was able to learn about the daily operation of a busy hospital department and gain insight into the role of the wider hospital team.

Spurred on by the experience I set out to organise further work experience, which included time spent in a renal transplant unit, a plastic surgery department in India, general practice and a district general hospital. I volunteered at a local care home on a weekly basis during term time and in my local hospital on Sunday mornings where I operated the tea trolley service. The variety of experience gained over the years preceding my application enabled me to make an informed decision to apply for Medicine.

At GCSE I achieved 9 A*s and 3 As. During my AS Levels I was awarded a Nuffield foundation bursary to work in the faculty of life sciences at Manchester University. This experience enabled me to gain insight into the world of Biomedical research.

I began writing my Personal Statement at the end of my AS Levels and booked the UKCAT for the end of August. Starting early meant I could review and revise the statement over time. I also made it a point to keep up to date with healthcare developments and news stories.

This is a snippet of my journey. I am currently studying clinical medicine at King's College London. Since starting medical school I have been involved in a range of activities and developed keen interests in medical education, leadership, quality improvement and patient safety. I was awarded the 2015 Sir John Ellis Prize by the Association for the Study of Medical Education for my work on the new King's College London MBBS curriculum 2020.

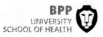

Medicine allows you to explore so much, I sincerely hope this book empowers you to look within your own journey and help you on your way to Medical School, and beyond.

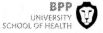

About the editors

Mr Gopal K Mahadev is a Consultant Surgeon with specialist interest in Breast Oncoplastic and General Surgery. He is a member of Court of Examiners for MRCS with the Royal College of Surgeons of England & FRCS Intercollegiate Board and is also involved in Quality Assurance of Assessments. He has worked as Senior Lecturer (Hon) in Medical Education and is a teacher, trainer, examiner and mentor for Medical Students and Surgical trainees as well as Consultants.

Matt Green BSc, MPhil has been mentoring students to successfully apply to Medical School for the last ten years and has extensive experience in guiding graduates through the process of successfully applying to normal and graduate entry programmes. One of Matt's passions is empowering individuals to follow their dream of pursuing a career in Medicine. This was a key motivator in producing this book, to help guide those individuals through the somewhat daunting steps of securing a place at Medical School.

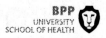

Chapter 1
Introduction

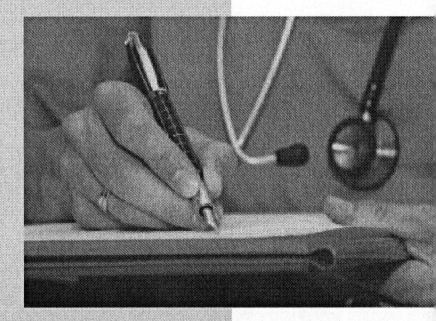

The most important question of all ...

Is Medicine for me?

This is the most important question in this book.

The best way to find out the answer is to try to gain as much exposure to as wide a range of healthcare environments as possible. This can be during work experience placements, in a voluntary capacity, or while undertaking a part-time job.

Speaking to healthcare professionals and asking questions about what their role involves is a great starting point.

We encourage you to visit the NHS Careers (www.healthcareers.nhs. uk) and A Taste of Medicine websites (www.tasteofmedicine.com). They both provide a good starting point to a career in healthcare.

Medical students and doctors come from all walks of life; there is no 'perfect' candidate for Medicine. Individuals have their own reasons for pursuing Medicine as a career and you should be certain that Medicine is what you really want to do.

Do not be pushed into the decision by other people.

As a doctor, you will need to be self-motivated, committed and willing to go the extra mile. Medicine is one of the most rewarding jobs in the world, but it is not for everyone. Once you're sure this is what you want, go for it!

We hope this book helps you to achieve your dream.

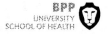

Work experience

Work experience is a vital part of the application process, both to ensure that Medicine is the right career path for you (which is most important), and to demonstrate commitment and passion to the admissions officers and interviewers.

Universities desire the following:

- Working as a healthcare assistant (HCA)
- Working as a carer for the elderly, people with disabilities or for children
- Working in a pharmacy
- Shadowing in hospitals
- Shadowing in GP surgeries
- Working in a university research laboratory

Sticking with a placement for several months shows genuine interest and commitment. You are also more likely to learn something about the attributes required to be a doctor, and how the healthcare system works, than if you flit from place to place.

You do not necessarily have to shadow a doctor on placement. Although this would be beneficial, you will learn a huge amount in the healthcare environment, working with any member of the healthcare team.

> ## Key Point:
> Consistency is key.

How do I get work experience for Medicine?

Medical work experience is a highly sought after opportunity. There are sometimes hundreds of students asking their local hospitals for placements. Here are some tips on getting a place:

1. Many hospitals operate placement waiting lists and these can be very long. As soon as you start to consider Medicine as a career, apply!

2. Make use of any contacts you know of who work in healthcare.

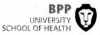

3. Take advantage of any experience that gives insight into a caring profession. This does not need to be hospital work experience or necessarily involve shadowing a doctor. Placements in schools or in a voluntary capacity are useful.

4. If a particular aspect of Medicine interests you, try contacting doctors who work in that field directly. Many have online profiles with their contact details. They will be much more likely to offer you a placement if you show genuine interest in what they do. You can draft a template letter or email to send to doctors who work in that area of Medicine. Below is an example:

Dear Mr/Ms/Mrs/Dr/Prof…

I hope this finds you well.

My name is…and I have just completed my AS Levels/GCSEs at…. I am very interested in pursuing a career in Medicine and came across your profile when researching the field that most appeals to me: Orthopaedics. Orthopaedics interests me as a keen sportsman, and I realise that the work you do with patients with sports injuries has a huge impact on their lives.

I would be most grateful if you could allow me to shadow you or someone in your department. I really would appreciate any opportunity you can offer.

Please find attached my CV for your consideration.

Kind regards,

Your name

School

Email Address and Phone Number

> ## *Key Point:*
> Although this may feel daunting, it requires little effort. You have nothing to lose, as there are only two outcomes – a reply or an ignored email/letter. If you don't ask, you don't get!

How long should I volunteer for?

Medical Schools are looking for committed individuals who show dedication and determination. A fortnight at the local care home in the summer holidays is unlikely to prove these attributes. Ideally, your voluntary experience should be long term over several months, on a regular basis. This can be as simple as a few hours serving coffee and tea to patients on Sunday mornings on a weekly or fortnightly basis.

It is advisable to keep a diary during all placements, be they paid or voluntary experiences. This helps you to draw upon your experiences in your Personal Statement and in your interview.

Key Point:

It is not the quantity of work experience you manage to obtain, but rather the quality, in terms of how you are able to reflect on your time.

Where should I volunteer?

There are numerous settings where you can volunteer your time, for example:

- GP surgeries
- Hospitals
- Pharmacies
- Hospices
- First aid charities, such as St John Ambulance
- Charity shops and events

You can also volunteer your time teaching or leading through:

- Sports coaching
- Tutoring younger peers
- Mentoring at school
- Helping at youth groups

Key Point:

The act of volunteering regardless of environment demonstrates that you are willing to help out and give up your time for others.

BPP
UNIVERSITY
SCHOOL OF HEALTH

How do you choose where to apply?

Open Days

Open Days (sometimes called Welcome or Visit Days) offer the best opportunity to see if a university is right for you.

You can get a real feel for the place, and have a good idea if you can see yourself being happy living and studying there for a number of years.

You can talk to current staff and most importantly students about the course, accommodation, and what it's like to live and study there.

There are also tours organised by the university around the accommodation, campus, sports facilities and libraries. Introductory talks are available for you and your parents/guardians to get a better idea about the course structure, extra-curricular activities on offer, financial and welfare support, and more.

Do not worry if you cannot make the official Open Day; it is still worthwhile visiting yourself because it lets you see if you think you could live and study there for five/six years. You can often arrange to have a current student take you around too.

Universities may offer online 'tours', or a forum to discuss with current students.

Where can I go with my grades?

It's important to be realistic; some universities may be out of reach with your predicted/achieved grades and/or admissions test results. You will have to research where you have the best chance of getting a place. Don't waste one of your four choices (applicants can only put down four out of their five UCAS choices as Medicine). It may be worthwhile doing the UKCAT earlier on so you know what your score is and can select appropriate Medical Schools based on this.

For up-to-date admissions information, contact universities directly, check their prospectus or visit their website. The Medical Schools Council website (www.medschools.ac.uk) also has useful information.

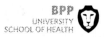

What is the course like / how will I be taught?

Medical Schools vary in their teaching style and method. The best way to find out about the course is to attend an Open Day and speak to current students; they can break the often-complicated structures provided in the prospectus into something you can understand and remember much more easily.

As highlighted above, you can research course structure on the Medical School website or in the university's prospectus.

Some important things to consider are: the weighting placed on Problem-Based Learning (PBL) compared to traditional lecture-based teaching; the possibility to intercalate in another degree; how anatomy is taught (dissection compared to prosection); and when patient contact first happens and how you are prepared for this.

Can I study for an intercalated degree?

Many Medical Schools allow students to take a year out to undertake an intercalated degree. This is an opportunity for students to pursue a subject outside of the standard medical curriculum. Some schools may allow students to intercalate at another university if they do not offer the subject they wish to study.

An advantage of undertaking such a degree is that it broadens your knowledge in an area of your choice. You will leave university with two degrees rather than one and this may enhance your career prospects. However, it is also important to take into account the extra year in education and the additional tuition fees and living costs. It is not necessary to do an intercalated degree just because your university offers one, and you should examine the pros and cons to inform your decision. There are many opportunities available for students to 'stand out' from the crowd during Medical School, such as through summer internships and university research projects.

Some students may also consider studying for a Masters (or even a Ph.D. degree) by taking an interruption from the medical programme, or moving to a joint programme within their university.

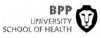

Rankings / League tables

Medical Schools are ranked every year based on recent graduate feedback. There are many criteria and questions used, and the findings are added together to come up with the 'best' universities. Some students like to use these as a starting point. One of the key results is student satisfaction, and this is something you can assess first-hand if you attend an Open Day.

You may find *Choosing a Medical School* by Alexander Young, Alexander Aquilina, Will Dougal, Thomas Judd and Matt Green, 2nd Edition published by BPP Learning Media, 2011 ISBN: 9781 4453 8150 3 a useful guide in selecting the best Medical School for you.

BPP
UNIVERSITY
SCHOOL OF HEALTH

Oxbridge

Oxford and Cambridge (Oxbridge) are two of the most prestigious and high-ranking universities in the world. There are some key things that make them stand out further from other universities.

Collegiate: Both Oxford and Cambridge are split into colleges, which makes for a close, community feel. Students belonging to a certain college will read a variety of subjects.

This arguably makes settling into university life easier, as every member of a certain college feels part of something bigger. It is also a great way to meet students from other courses. The other benefit is that you develop a good relationship with tutors and pastoral/support staff.

Tutorials/supervisions: Oxford has tutorials; Cambridge has supervisions. These are small group classes, where you will be thoroughly challenged. You have regular individual attention and feedback will be personal. You will be both challenged and supported by a member of staff who will learn a lot about you. Clearly this style of learning/teaching requires a large amount of preparatory study.

Oxbridge offers a unique student experience and the teaching is first-class. However, it is not for everyone. As highlighted above, it is important to visit universities on Open Days (perhaps more so for Oxbridge, because they are so unique). Talk to staff and students to get a good insight into student life.

Remember you have to sit the BioMedical Admissions Test (BMAT) to apply to Oxbridge, and you can only apply to either Oxford or Cambridge, not both.

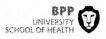

Applying to Medical Schools

A useful resource is the British Medical Association's Guide for Studying Medicine:

http://bma.org.uk/developing-your-career/becoming-a-doctor/entry-to-medical-school

The Student British Medical Journal (sBMJ), a great resource to keep up to date with topical medical issues, provides a Med School Selector tool: http://medschoolselector.student.bmj.com/#/home – which matches your grades to Medical School entry criteria so you can choose the right course for you.

When is the deadline for applying to Medical School?

The deadline for applying via the Universities and Colleges Admissions Service (UCAS) is 15th October. However, preparation should begin long before to show Admissions Tutors that you have the commitment Medicine demands. More importantly, before you apply you should have a real understanding of what Medicine entails and firmly believe that Medicine is what you really want to do.

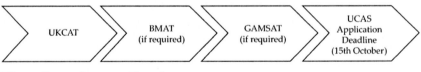

Flowchart for application process

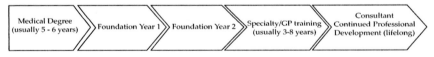

Flowchart from now to consultant

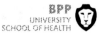

Can I apply to study Medicine without a background in science?

There are a number of options available for individuals with a non-science background who wish to study Medicine. Some universities have slightly longer foundation programmes to ensure all applicants have the prior knowledge required to study Medicine. It is worth asking each Medical School about such schemes, researching their entry requirements, consulting Medical School websites and reading prospectuses.

Do I need to know what type of doctor I want to be before Medical School?

No. For many medical students in their late teenage years, making the decision to apply to study Medicine is already a big one. Thus, being asked to choose what type of doctor you want to be is extremely difficult. Some may have an idea about what they would like to specialise in. In reality, however, as you gain exposure to the many specialities during your education and training years, you are likely to change your mind a number of times. You should keep an open mind and not discount any career options.

Studying Medicine abroad

With high tuition fees and increasing competition in the UK, many students are looking abroad for their medical studies. It is important to note, however, that to practise in the UK you must ensure the medical degree is recognised by the General Medical Council (GMC). There are some overseas Medical Schools that will allow you to subsequently undertake NHS foundation training after graduating. Always verify your choice of institution with the GMC before applying to the course.

There are a number of online communities that have discussions on Medical Schools popular amongst students from the UK. Try speaking to current students at foreign universities for their views on the course and life abroad.

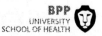

Some useful links:

- A Star Future http://www.astarfuture.co.uk/study_medicine_abroad.html
- The Student Room (TSR) http://www.thestudentroom.co.uk/forum.php
- GMC www.gmc-uk.org

Chapter 2
Admissions Tests

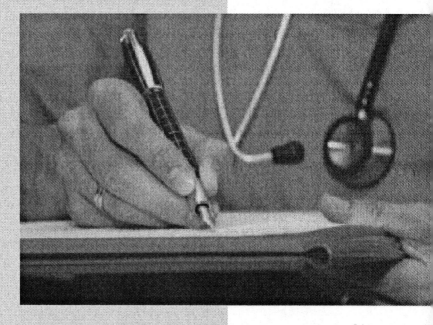

UKCAT

What is the UKCAT?

The UK Clinical Aptitude Test (UKCAT) is a computer-based exam used by a consortium of Medical Schools in the UK in their admissions process (www.ukcat.ac.uk/about-the-test/who-should-take-the-test/).

At the time of writing, you have to take the UKCAT between the beginning of July and the beginning of October.

How can I prepare for the UKCAT?

As with any test, practice is important. The UKCAT is different to the average public examinations you will have sat before. It is completed on a computer in an official test centre, similar to how the driving theory test is administered.

1. The UKCAT website provides important up-to-date information about the test along with sample tests. These are the only official resources available. You can get used to the computer system using these sample tests.

2. There are a number of books available for UKCAT practice. Although these are not officially endorsed, they allow students to build confidence and become accustomed to the format and content. If you are struggling to develop strategies or are intimidated by questions, it may be worthwhile working through some practice books.

3. Along with books, there are various UKCAT courses available. Once again, these are not formally endorsed, and may be expensive. Ask friends, your school or forums for recommendations.

The UKCAT is split into five sections:

1. Verbal Reasoning
2. Quantitative Reasoning
3. Abstract Reasoning
4. Decision Analysis
5. Situational Judgement

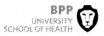

The UKCAT for Special Educational Needs (UKCATSEN) is available for those that are entitled to additional time in public examinations due to a medical condition.

Make sure you reschedule your UKCAT to a later date if you are unwell.

Further information can be found on the UKCAT website: www. ukcat.ac.uk

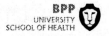

BMAT

What is the BMAT?

The BioMedical Admissions Test (BMAT) is a two-hour, pen-and-paper test divided into three sections:

1. Aptitude and Skills
2. Scientific Knowledge and Applications
3. Writing Task

A few universities in the UK require the BMAT. Currently, University College London, Imperial College London, Brighton and Sussex, University of Leeds, Lancaster, Oxford and the Cambridge Medical Schools use the test in their selection process.

How can I prepare for the BMAT?

The BMAT website has some official resources to practise from.

The only official book is entitled *Preparing for the BMAT* and can be found here – http://www.pearsonschoolsandfecolleges. co.uk/Secondary/Science/16OtherSciences/PreparingfortheBMAT/ PreparingfortheBMAT.aspx

There is also an Assumed Knowledge Guide on the BMAT website. This is essential reading!

Further information can be found on the BMAT website:

http://www.admissionstestingservice.org/for-test-takers/bmat/ about-bmat/

There are also a number of revision books which include practice tests and explanations to help you prepare for the BMAT. We recommend: *Succeeding in the Biomedical Admissions Test (BMAT)* by Matt Green and Nicola Hawley, published by BPP Learning Media, 2012. ISBN 9781 4453 8164 0

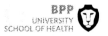

General advice for admissions tests

Registration: Register in plenty of time!

Weeks before: Get into a good sleeping pattern. Do your exam practice, using books, online resources and courses (if you want to). It's worthwhile reading broadsheets regularly to ensure your English is at a high standard (if you read health news stories you'll be better prepared for your interviews too!). Ensure your mental maths is at a proficient level. Work through GCSE-level past papers and try cutting their time limit in half. If you need any help, BBC Bitesize is a good resource. Try to do plenty of exercise; exercising outside is good for getting a bit of fresh air.

Night before: Ensure you get a good night's sleep before your exam. Try to do something you enjoy that will calm you before bed (light exercise and a shower/bath is a good bet). Make sure you have all of the required documents looked out, eg a map for the test centre location, any travel tickets, your exam booking confirmation, any ID required, and any equipment you might need (glasses/contacts, pencils/pens etc).

Eat a good breakfast (and lunch): Have a filling breakfast with lots of slow-release carbohydrates. The exams all last a long time so you need to ensure your brain has all the energy it needs. If you can stomach it, have some glucose tablets before you start for a good energy spike.

Test centre journey: As with interviews, make sure you know where you're going and leave in plenty of time! If you can, do a practice run beforehand which will ease your nerves on the big day.

Take a break: Take a few seconds periodically to have a quick stretch and get a good breath in to maintain good oxygen levels to your brain, and to help combat tiredness.

Question triage: Don't spend too much time on one hard question. Ensure you complete all questions – even if this means putting an educated guess down before the time limit is up.

If things don't go so well: Don't panic! This is just one part of your application process. Some Medical Schools place more emphasis on UKCAT scores than others. Contact Medical Schools directly to find out how they use UKCAT in their selection process.

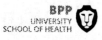

Graduate Entry Medicine

Medicine for graduates and mature students

The application process for Graduate Entry Medicine (GEM) varies at each Medical School. It may be the case that those with science degrees can apply for accelerated four-year programmes. There are limited places for these graduate entry courses and competition is very high. It is always worth checking with each school if they have a graduate/mature entry programme and how it operates.

A number of Medical Schools allow graduates to apply through UCAS as an undergraduate.

Some Medical Schools may require graduate students to undertake the GAMSAT (see below). At the time of writing, these include Cardiff, Exeter, Liverpool, Nottingham, Plymouth (Peninsula), St George's and Swansea.

More information regarding GEM can be found at the below links:

- www.medschools.ac.uk/students/courses/pages/graduate.aspx (lists all UK Medical Schools currently offering the accelerated four-year GEM course)
- www.medicalcareers.nhs.uk/considering_Medicine/graduate_entry_programme.aspx (further information for those considering GEM)

What is the GAMSAT?

The Graduate (Australian) Medical School Admissions Test (GAMSAT) is a test used to differentiate graduate applicants.

The GAMSAT is split into three sections:

1. Reasoning in Humanities and Social Sciences
2. Written Communication
3. Reasoning in Biological and Physical Sciences

The GAMSAT coordinators release new Information booklets every year, so check on the website that the GAMSAT remains the same.

There is only one chance each year to sit the GAMSAT. Ensure you register in good time and don't miss the day!

ACER produces the only official GAMSAT preparation material. Find this and further information via the GAMSAT website: http:// gamsat.acer.edu.au/gamsat-uk

Personal Statement

The Personal Statement is a vital part of your application to study Medicine and thus key to a successful application. Writing one requires genuine insight, patience and determination. It is your opportunity to showcase yourself in the best possible way to each Medical School. In many cases, your Personal Statement will also set the tone to any interviews, so it is important that you're able to discuss in detail anything that you have written.

What is the Personal Statement?

The Personal Statement is the most important part of your UCAS Application. You have 47 lines (including blank lines) and/or 4,000 characters (whichever comes first) to tell universities why they should offer you a place. Most students applying to study Medicine will have similar grades and many will have positions of responsibility at their school/college (Head Boy/Girl or Prefect). The Personal Statement is your chance to shine, show what you've learnt from your work experience, what you can bring to the university and why you know Medicine is right for you.

There is no perfect Personal Statement and, as cliché as it sounds, it is something which is unique to you as it reflects your journey to becoming a doctor. It should include:

- Your ambition to study Medicine

- Why you think you possess the qualities a good doctor needs

- Any experiences you have gained in order to inform your decision

- Extra-curricular activities you are involved in and positions of responsibility you hold

When writing it is necessary to reflect as well as describe. Reflection is your chance to relate experiences to yourself and to Medicine as a future career.

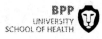

A good place to start is by writing down everything you have done that has any relevance to studying Medicine.

- School subjects

- Books you have read or journals you read

- Writing or research you have done: *Young Scientists' Journal* (www.ysjournal.com), *Lancet Student* (www.thelancetstudent. com) and *TMS* (www.themedicalstudent.co.uk) may accept your writing for publication

- Work experience/shadowing placements

- Voluntary or paid work in the medical world

- Conferences, courses or lectures you have attended

- Part-time jobs

- Charity and voluntary work

- Sports, music and other extra-curricular activities

- Positions you hold at school, eg Prefect status, peer mentoring, sports captain etc

- Duke of Edinburgh, and Young Enterprise experiences

- Any travelling you have done

- Hobbies and interests (musical instruments you play, languages you speak …)

Use UCAS's Personal Statement Worksheet to get all of the key information down on paper: http://www.ucas.com/sites/default/files/personal-statement-worksheet.pdf

It's easier to cut down a long Personal Statement than build up a short one, so get everything relevant down and only take things out if you need to.

If you're applying for deferred entry it's important that you explain why! Say what you plan to do, why, and how this will be of benefit to your future as a medical student and ultimately as a doctor. Perhaps you plan to work to raise money to fund your studies, maybe you want to learn a language, or maybe you want to travel.

It is worthwhile having a look at some exemplar Personal Statements to get an idea of how students put their passion across, and some

BPP
UNIVERSITY
SCHOOL OF HEALTH

good ways of structuring the Statement. Your school may be able to provide you with some examples, or you can research online. Alternatively you can use books written to help you with your Personal Statement. We have included our successful Personal Statements to give you some ideas. Please be aware, however, that plagiarism will be identified by UCAS.

Some important things to address and display:

- Conscientious and hard-working nature
- Empathy, care and compassion
- Ability to cope with stress and high work demands
- Communication skills
- Ability to work with others (as a team member and as a leader)
- Desire and passion for Medicine, with an insight into the challenges and positives of the degree and vocation
- Understanding of the importance of a good work-life balance

Some useful tips and advice:

- Have strong opening and concluding sentences, to ensure a reader is keen to continue and that you leave a memorable impression
- Don't start every sentence with 'I'
- Only use words you actually use otherwise it won't sound natural
- Don't repeat things they can get from your UCAS form, eg grades
- Formatting (bold, italics or underlining) does not appear on the end product

It's useful to research each of the universities you are applying to, as they often spell out what they want the Personal Statement to show. Ensure you meet all of the targets set by every university you're planning to apply to.

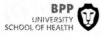

Ensure you don't tailor your Personal Statement solely to your top choice (eg Oxbridge) because other universities will disregard your application if you talk about wanting to study in tutorials/ supervisions.

Ask your friends and family members to check through your Personal Statement initially. They may be able to give you some feedback to improve your early drafts.

It is a good idea to ask an English teacher if you have access to one to double-check your grammar and general writing structure.

After you have worked through several drafts and feel it's as good as you can get it, give your Statement to a teacher who deals with UCAS, or to a healthcare professional. Their analysis will be invaluable.

Visit UCAS's site for some hints and tips: www.ucas.com/how-it-all-works/undergraduate/filling-your-application/your-personal-statement

---

Key Points:

- Start planning and improving your Personal Statement early

- Do not plagiarise

- Do not fabricate anything

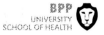

Example Personal Statements

Example 1

My ambition to study Medicine arises from my keen interest in the sciences, especially in the human body. I am fascinated by medical treatments and it is my desire to work with people from all walks of life to improve their wellbeing.

To gain insight and determine my suitability for Medicine I organised various work experience placements, the first of which was in Nuclear Medicine at Manchester Royal Infirmary (MRI) in July 2007. It was intriguing to discover how radioisotope scans were used in determining organ functions. This made me realise the diversity of Medicine. At the MRI Renal Unit in Summer 2008 I was able to gain an understanding of the work of multidisciplinary teams and able to fully appreciate how different members contributed to the overall care of patients. It was encouraging to see patients improving post-transplantation and adapting to immunosuppressant regimens. I developed an understanding of the essential qualities of a good doctor such as knowledge, honesty, a sense of humour, and seeing patients as individuals and not just symptoms.

Another interesting placement was at the Apollo Hospital (India) in April 2009 where it was inspiring to observe surgical procedures such as the removal of a cancerous growth as well as being exposed to a foreign healthcare environment.

Since October 2008, I have volunteered weekly at Southbank nursing home. I find time spent here most valuable as it gives me insight into traumas associated with terminal illness, death, age related conditions and diseases such as senile dementia. It taught me and constantly reminds me that Medicine is as much about caring as it is about curing. In addition, volunteering at Trafford General Hospital has taught me the criticality of a cleanliness culture in fighting infection and general ward duties in patient care. In July 2009, I was given the opportunity at this hospital of a medical taster course. Shadowing consultants and junior doctors working under pressure often with a lack of resources has enabled me to appreciate the importance of hard work, organisation and communication in a doctor–patient relationship.

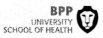
BPP
UNIVERSITY
SCHOOL OF HEALTH

I competed for and was awarded a four-week Nuffield Scholarship at the Faculty of Life Sciences at Manchester University. Here I worked with doctorate students conducting experiments using advanced techniques and realised the importance of dedication in achieving medical progress. I was interested by platelet-derived growth factor and its use in embryogenesis and I wrote a report on this research which was selected for a Gold Crest Award. To develop my independent learning skills I studied for the Open University module 'Molecules, Medicines and Drugs'; and also prepared a paper on stem cells which was published online.

Alongside Academia, I lead a music group in which I play the drums. Our much rehearsed 'unique' acts have been selected for many charitable events including playing at Trafalgar Square, European Capital of Culture Finale show and Water Aid. I enjoy debating, whether as President of my school Hindu Society or Co-president of the School Medical Society. I improved my public speaking by training and obtained a distinction at LAMDA grade 8. I believe in community participation and am a founding team leader of the Trafford Vinvolved Action team where I regularly work for causes such as Cancer Research and Henshaws. I also learnt sign language which has allowed me to work with the deaf.

Having played for the school hockey team since Year 7, I have learned the value of team spirit and commitment. I also enjoyed developing my leadership skills whilst pursuing my Duke of Edinburgh Gold Award and my aspiration now is to climb Mt. Kilimanjaro for charity.

In conclusion, I am committed to be part of the positive impact Medicine has on society and have the enthusiasm, determination and the attributes to take on the challenges of studying Medicine and make a real contribution as a doctor.

Example 2

Hearing a car crash into my father when we were out cycling was sickening. Not knowing how to help was worse. I therefore enrolled on a First Aid course, which started me on the path towards a medical career. Besides providing an opportunity to study the complexities of the human body, Medicine offers a platform to make a difference to society. I want to be part of this.

To appreciate what it takes, I've experienced a variety of medical settings: a surgical firm at Leighton Hospital, dialysis in Spain, a GP surgery, and a hospice. The variety of illnesses captured my imagination. It felt as if each doctor was a detective – gathering information from the body's signs and patient's symptoms to reach a diagnosis. Fascinating as this was, I began to experience how patients cope with disease and to understand the importance of seeing the individual behind the illness. Observing professionals managing each situation with the utmost compassion was inspiring. With the same compassion, and maturity, I could empathise with patients receiving bad news. A personal highlight was an MDT meeting, which emphasised the importance of teamwork. Listening to experts from differing specialties give their unique insight into each case was fantastic.

My A Levels have provided a strong academic foundation. Chemistry improved my problem-solving skills, whereas Biology introduced me to the captivating world of Human Biology. In Year 12 I achieved A* in Maths, showing I have the focus needed for success in higher education. Recognising the importance of Statistics when evaluating research, I took S2 and S3 in a Further Maths AS. To understand more about Medicine, I studied 'Molecules, medicines and drugs' with the OU, demonstrating independent learning. I've attended interesting lectures, including 'Doctors in the Dock', which highlighted the legal consequences of malpractice. My ECDL will be useful, as my placements have shown how crucial IT skills are in modern Medicine.

As Head Boy my organisational and time-management skills developed, as I had to balance this responsibility with my studies and extra-curricular activities. I've seen first-hand how health professionals put these skills into action. Through school I helped at a care home, which gave me an insight into care of the elderly: how being there for someone makes a real difference. In 6th Form I was also involved in a fundraising group, set up in memory of a former pupil. We raised

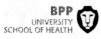

money for The Christie Hospital and were delighted to be recognised with a Diana Award.

My activities out of school have stressed the importance of committing myself to something in order to achieve it. This is certainly true of the D of E Scheme, which has reinforced the value of teamwork, determination and commitment. I've been very fortunate to travel extensively: from the Far East to South America. Whilst on expedition in Ecuador, summiting Cotopaxi (19,347 ft) in extreme conditions showed I have the perseverance to achieve anything! As the only Spanish speaker in the group my leadership and communication skills flourished.

Having witnessed how exhausting a medical career can be, I've pushed myself to ensure I have the stamina required. I've also seen the need for an escape from this demanding vocation. Mine is cycling; I enjoy riding to raise money for health-related causes.

I see my gap year as a time to develop my strengths and further explore Medicine. I'm therefore involved with St John Ambulance and the Samaritans, which allow me to interact directly with people in need. Having been active in Scouting for 12 years, and a volunteer at Beavers for almost 3, I'm now training to become a Leader. I plan to work and save money to travel next summer, to gain further independence before university.

Medicine is a rewarding career that truly matters in society. Whilst researching the course my passion has only intensified. This is what I want to do for the rest of my life.

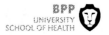

Example 3

Prior to losing consciousness during an episode of my Wolff-Parkinson-White syndrome I saw the look of anguish on my mum's face. When I recovered, her face was full of joy and relief. Realising that doctors caused this dramatic change had a profound effect on me.

This was the spark that first got me interested in Medicine.

This was further reinforced as a student at Altrincham Grammar School. My inquisitiveness into complex intricacies of the human body was developed and nurtured by teachers, who advised me and encouraged my interest in Biology. Learning about the astounding aspects of human anatomy and numerous ways of its working captures my imagination.

As a Deputy Head Boy of school and head of the Medical Society, I had the responsibility to work with other students and organise formal and social events as well as arrange weekly meetings thus improving my organisational skills.

Being Captain of both football and basketball teams improved my ability to work effectively in a team as well as develop my leadership skills. Being an assistant coach for an U12 football team has given me the responsibility to teach and train children. Currently, I'm training to attain a Level 1 coaching badge which will enable me to coach a team on my own, as well as provide me with First Aid and leadership skills.

I was a member of Chad's challenges, a fundraising group for The Christie's Cancer Centre. This, I felt, was a very rewarding experience as our efforts could change someone's life.

Wanting to learn and understand more about Medicine, I undertook work experience enthusiastically both in a Paediatric Ward and a pharmacy. Working at a pharmacy was a unique experience. This not only gave me an insight into patient aftercare and drug impact but also improved my communication skills as I built up a rapport with patients. The work experience on the Paediatric Ward at Stepping Hill Hospital was fantastic. Interacting with children, observing the teamwork and trying to understand the doctors' techniques of intervention had a tremendous impact on me. Witnessing the work in the neo-natal unit was an incredible experience and made me realise what a medical marvel an incubator is!

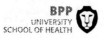

In addition, I volunteered at a care home for a year. I enjoyed talking to the residents, assisted them with their daily routines and just being there for them. Although challenging, I was able to overcome many barriers thus enabling me to be more confident in my abilities.

Currently, during my gap year I am undertaking work experience at Leighton Hospital, Crewe. My experiences so far have been exceptional, reinforcing my commitment to undertake Medicine as a career. I had the opportunity to attend clinics, both new and follow up, gained insight into assessment and see results of surgery. Being in an operating theatre, I have been fortunate to see surgery such as tumour removal, breast reconstruction and endoscopies.

Furthermore, I now understand better the impact treatment has on a patient's life. Attending the MDT meetings showed me the teamwork and decision-making skills needed as a doctor. It is impressive how expertise from various specialities, working together, benefit the patients. The interaction and discussion among the experts was fascinating. I want to be part of all this!

Listening to many of the doctors' experiences, I am convinced that I am making the right choice to undertake a medical career. I sincerely feel that I have the qualities of care, compassion, dedication and perseverance, to see a job completed. I am sure to develop them further as I gain experience.

Studying Medicine will allow me to accomplish my passion to help people; the satisfaction gained from finding, treating and hopefully curing diseases must be phenomenal. As a hard-working and caring person I am confident that I can undertake the vigorous and rewarding journey of studying Medicine.

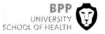

Example 4

My inspiration to study Medicine came when I had a successful operation on a broken cheekbone. The maxillofacial surgery prevented me from having a permanent facial disfiguration. This left me with great admiration for the medical profession and a passion to help others as they had helped me. Studying Medicine will provide the perfect mix as it links my fascination for human biology with my desire to work with people in a caring capacity in the community. It will present the ideal combination of utilising my ability to work well in a team with strong leadership skills and effective communication with peers. A career in Medicine will give me new challenges every day while also being rewarding, in seeing the improvement of patients via the application of various treatments and care. As a very self-motivated person, shown in my completion of the Open University course 'Molecules, Medicine and Drugs', I will keep acquainted with the lifelong learning process that is modern Medicine.

My fascination with Medicine led me to undertake shadowing at Bolton Hospital in Thoracic Medicine and South Manchester University Hospital's Vascular Medicine. This gave me a real insight into what being a doctor entails. Observing an angioplasty reinforced how essential teamwork is, with the surgical team working in harmony to operate on the patient. Care and compassion shown to patients were absolutely compelling and reaffirmed my commitment to Medicine. During my gap year I am currently doing work experience at Leighton Hospital as an observer in clinics, endoscopies, surgery and MDT meetings. The MDT meetings have highlighted the importance of communication between various specialities. To gain experience and understanding, I undertook weekly volunteer work at Heathside Residential Home for the Elderly. This involved entertaining as well as looking after the needs of the elderly residents. This was an invaluable experience for me, demonstrating that comforting patients is essential, especially those with incurable diseases such as Alzheimer's and cancer.

As Deputy Head Boy of my school, and Prefect of the Amnesty International Society, I had the responsibility of organising prefects, attending school events and running meetings. Being a member of the school rugby team taught me to be a good team player, and in my role as a Young Enterprise team director I learnt to be an effective and motivational leader. I am nearing completion of my Duke of Edinburgh

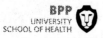

Gold Award that has required a lot of commitment. As a self-starter, I have learnt various musical instruments including bass and guitar. My part-time job as an assistant at my local pharmacy has been extremely useful in developing my interpersonal and communication skills, as well as establishing a good rapport with patients. Being active in my local community I raised money for 'Chad's Challenges', a cancer charity for The Christie Cancer Centre. For my contribution I was awarded the 'Diana Certificate of Excellence'. I organised and managed numerous events for the charity, including a very successful rock music night at my school, which helped to raise money. I'm also currently helping run a youth club. This has given me greater understanding of engaging with children. Simultaneously I am earning money to travel later in my gap year, which will help me achieve greater independence prior to university. My interest in science and Medicine means that I keep up to date with the latest medical and scientific issues through my reading of 'Student BMJ' and 'New Scientist'.

My work experience and voluntary work have strengthened my resolve to study Medicine, and my extra-curricular activities show I have the skills and qualities needed. I am confident that given the opportunity I will fulfil my dream and become a good doctor.

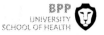

Interviews

Most Medical Schools interview prospective students. Don't be worried if you haven't heard from the universities you have applied to. No news is good news; they are still considering your application.

How should I prepare for my interview?

However obvious this sounds – know your Personal Statement inside out. The worst scenario is when the interviewer asks the candidate a question about their Personal Statement and they are left dumbfounded.

The interview can focus on any aspect of your Personal Statement. It doesn't matter if you only spent 25 minutes in the renal transplant ward. Be prepared for a question on the transplant process.

After writing your Personal Statement, research everything that could potentially be questioned from those 4,000 characters. Keeping a diary during work experience can help you describe and reflect on your experiences, and anecdotes make your interview stand out.

Think critically about your Personal Statement. You could ask someone to come up with challenging questions from the content.

Keep abreast of recent changes in the medical world. You should to be able to talk about recent health news stories, giving a brief overview and your views on the matter.

Another thing to do before interview is to research the course and the university itself. You have to know how the course is structured – what you'll be taught and how, and what sets it apart from other Medical Schools.

Key Points:

- Know your Personal Statement inside out

- Keep up to date with recent health news

- Understand how and what you will be taught at each university

---

Recommended reading

We have found the following books to be of great interest:

- *Medical Ethics: A Very Short Introduction* (Tony Hope)
- *The Emperor of All Maladies* (Siddhartha Mukherjee)
- *The Rise and Fall of Modern Medicine* (James Le Fanu)
- *Trust Me, I'm a Junior Doctor* (Max Pemberton)
- *Medicine's 10 Greatest Discoveries* (Meyer Friedman and Gerald W Friedland)

We have also found the following resources to be extremely useful:

- *Student BMJ*
- *New Scientist*
- BBC Health
- Ted.com
- GMC Student News (http://www.gmc-uk.org/information_for_you/student_gmc_news.asp)

Keep a folder and collect anything in the general press or in medical journals that takes your interest. Refer back to these from time to time. This will ensure you keep abreast of any changes in the medical world, and the folder offers an archive for you to refer back to before your interviews.

Interview practice

It is important to practise your interview technique before the real thing. You can ask friends and family members if they would be willing to help you out to start with. Once you are used to the feel of speaking about and selling yourself, you should ask someone you don't know to conduct the interview. If you are a school student, a senior teacher is a good idea. Alternatively, if there are other nearby schools or colleges you could set up an exchange if teachers are willing: you can get interviewed at their college and their students come to your school and get interviewed by a member of your college's staff.

Ask for feedback from these interviews, and record their advice and suggestions.

You will soon be much more comfortable and will be able to concentrate on what you're saying rather than how it feels to sell yourself in front of others.

After practising with friends, family and teachers it would be a good idea to practise with fellow applicants if you know any. You will know which questions you find difficult – be mean to each other!

Once you feel comfortable with the general process, see if someone you find intimidating is willing to quiz you! This will really help your nerves when it comes to the real thing.

Another thing that can be helpful is to video yourself, and check that you don't fidget, which can be distracting for listeners.

Confidence

Confidence is key to a successful interview. You have a great opportunity to show the interviewers how you cope in high-pressure situations.

You should be confident: the Medical School has offered you an interview, so they are interested in **you**, and see potential in **you**.

Confidence will come with practice, so be proactive and ask for help!

There are a couple of techniques which may help:

Positive Visualisation: Every time you think about your interview, imagine yourself having the 'perfect' interview. You arrive on time, are greeted by the panel and you smile and give them a confident handshake. You are asked questions that you have practised in the past and give well-structured and succinct answers. They ask some trickier questions but you think logically and answer calmly. They are interested in your responses and your enthusiasm and passion are evident. You thank them for their time, shake hands and leave with a big smile on your face.

Emotional Anchoring: Whenever you are feeling happy, calm and relaxed in the run up to your interview, rub your finger and thumb together. If you build up an 'emotional anchor', when you do this same action in your interview you should feel the same again, which will have a great calming effect and let your confidence shine through. You could try doing this 'anchoring' after your positive visualisation.

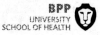

You can show the interview panel you are confident as soon as you walk into the room. Give them all a firm handshake, smile and look them in the eye. When you are asked to take a seat, sit up straight and maintain eye contact with the interviewers. This could be difficult if there are multiple interviewers so focus on the person who is talking to you. When answering questions make sure to smile, and aim for eye contact the majority of the time.

Note. If you find it hard to look the examiner in the eye a little tip is to look at the bridge of their nose; they won't be able to tell the difference.

Rushing into your answer is not a sign of confidence; don't be afraid to take a moment to think about your answer and then reply.

Your body language is also a big giveaway about your confidence. Make sure you have 'open body language'. Turn and face your body towards the interviewer and have your arms uncrossed. Hand movements are also useful when answering questions, as you can emphasise points and it stops you fidgeting with them, giving an air of confidence and enthusiasm. Try not to touch your face or hair, as this suggests nervousness and uncertainty. Nod your head to show you are paying attention.

When you go for interview practice you can ask the 'interviewer' how you can improve your body language and eye contact. Heed their advice and put it into practice!

Finally, on completion of the interview shake hands, thank the panel for their time and smile. You've done your best!

We have explained a couple of useful techniques below, which will help you to leave a great impression on the interview panel.

The 'Rule of three'

This is a simple yet effective technique with which you can structure any answer. It simply means that you have to split your response into three parts. This not only makes it easy for you to organise and communicate your thoughts, but also makes it more manageable for the interview panel to absorb.

For example, when answering: 'What makes a good doctor?'

You could break down your answer into the following:

- Care and compassion
- 'People skills' (leader/manager, effective communicator, team player)
- Makes patients feel comfortable (through confidence, ability and knowledge, and empathy)

This technique means you can have a structured response ready in your mind, which you can then verbalise to the panel, meaning your answers do not sound rehearsed, but remain clear and concise.

Anecdotes

Anecdotes allow you to put a personal touch on your interview. They show that you were not merely a passive 'passenger' during your work experience, and that you got involved and interacted with the patients you met. Anecdotes are memorable for interviewers, and ensure a break in monotony for them. It's much better to include your own stories than to simply blurt out a 'textbook' answer.

'Oddball' questions

Be prepared for occasional unconventional questions, which are used to test your thought process. Stay calm and think things through before rushing into providing a bad answer. Make sure your answer is concise so that you don't lose your interviewers' attention.

- Don't panic
- Think logically
- Be concise

One more sleep!

It's finally arrived, one more sleep until your interview.

Ensure you have all that you need for your interview ready: a map of the interview location, any travel tickets, any ID required, and (if required) exam certificates, evidence of work experience, and medical forms.

BPP
UNIVERSITY
SCHOOL OF HEALTH

You can have a quick look over your Personal Statement, your BMAT essay (if applicable), the prospectus and a look on BBC Health. However, the night before is not a time to start cramming! Once you've had a quick look over these, relax.

Go for a run, listen to some music or watch a comedy. Just do something you enjoy that will calm your nerves.

Don't have a heavy meal (or drink a lot of coffee!) that could make sleep troublesome. Get a good night's sleep, and wake up early. Have a leisurely breakfast and a leisurely journey to the interview centre – don't rush and keep your cool.

This is it – **good luck!**

Key Points:

- Practice is key
- Be confident
- Use the 'rule of three' to keep answers concise
- Use anecdotes to make your interview memorable

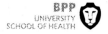

Chapter 3
Need to know

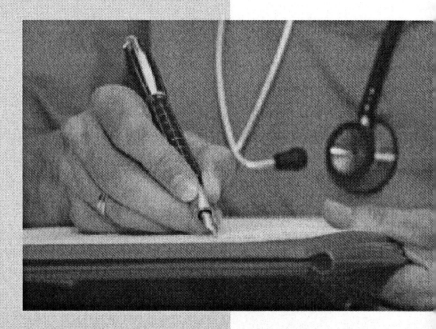

We have collated 'need to know' information for applying to Medical School (and beyond...). We start with your 'Journey from application to qualification', with information on the UCAS process and terms you have to be aware of. We then move on to 'Organisations and policies'; looking at the NHS, governing bodies and more. 'Ethics and law' is the next section, looking at the legal requirements and arguments for and against some key issues. We finish with a look at 'Medical conditions and disease processes', which are important to be aware of, especially if you mention them in your Personal Statement.

Journey from application to qualification

UKCAT

The **UK Clinical Aptitude Test** is a test for entry to certain Medical Schools in the UK. The majority of Medical Schools employ this test to aid selection. See page 14 for more information.

BMAT

A few universities in the UK administer the **BioMedical Admission Test**. Currently, University College London, Imperial College London, Brighton and Sussex, Leeds, Lancaster, Oxford and Cambridge use this test in their selection process (January 2016). See page 16 for more information.

GAMSAT

The GAMSAT is the Graduate Entry Medicine (GEM) equivalent of the UKCAT/BMAT. It tests basic science knowledge, critical thinking, problem solving and writing skills. See page 18 for more information.

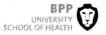

Intercalations

Many Medical Schools offer a 'sandwich' degree (in a year) to those students who show the required proficiency for this level of study and commitment.

Electives

Electives provide an opportunity to study and learn away from your Medical School. Many students go abroad during their clinical years for 6–12 weeks, to experience Medicine in a different setting. The opportunities are endless and need not be 'clinical' – research and education posts are also available. Although many students go abroad, a number stay in the UK.

Postgraduate training

Training to become a GP or Consultant takes differing amounts of time, but all Medicine graduates wishing to become a doctor must first complete two years of training as a 'Foundation/Junior Doctor'. In the first year (FY1), you will rotate through three or four jobs in different specialities. The year builds upon the training and skills learnt as an undergraduate and upon completion you will be fully registered with the General Medical Council (GMC). In the second year (FY2), you will do further posts in different specialities and build upon competencies learnt in the first year. At this stage you will be required to make decisions on your future career path.

The next stage to becoming a GP or Consultant, following your two years as a Foundation Doctor, is to become a 'Specialist Registrar'. Those wishing to become a GP currently do three years in general practice, and those wishing to become a Consultant will do a minimum of six years in a hospital speciality. Specialist Registrars will take part in structured training programmes directly after their completion as a Foundation Doctor.

Overall, this means that following your undergraduate training you must complete a minimum of a further eight years' training to become a Consultant and five years to become a GP.

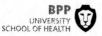

UCAS

To apply to UK universities, you must use UCAS, the Universities and Colleges Application Service. You have to complete an application form, which involves personal details, educational history and achievements, and your Personal Statement. The application deadline is 15th October, for entry in the autumn of the following year.

Organisations and policies

NHS

The NHS was set up through the 'National Health Service Act 1946'. Prior to this people had to pay for treatment, with healthcare only occasionally being available for free from charity and teaching hospitals.

The 'National Insurance Act 1911' ensured that in exchange for contributions from their paycheck, workers were entitled to medical care, but not necessarily to the drugs needed. There was a consensus prior to World War II that reform was needed with dependants also receiving health insurance, and that different types of hospitals should be integrated. However, due to WWII, no action was taken.

The post-war reconstruction gave an opportunity, which might not have been possible in peacetime, for the NHS to be set up. The 'Beveridge Report' of 1942 identified disease as being one of the 'Five Great Evils' as it prevented men from working and therefore caused financial problems. The report gained bipartisan support as well as massive public support. In 1945, following Labour's election victory, multiple social policies, known as the 'Welfare State', were introduced, including the 'National Health Service Act 1946'.

The NHS was finally launched on 5 July 1948 with three core principles:

- To meet the needs of everybody
- To be free at the point of delivery
- To be based on clinical need, not ability to pay

MHRA

The **Medicines & Healthcare products Regulatory Agency** (MHRA) regulates the safety of the medicines and medical devices used in the UK.

GMC

The **General Medical Council** (GMC) is a body that has a statutory duty in maintaining the registration of medical practitioners within the UK.

The main roles that the GMC undertakes are:

- Registering doctors to practise with provisional or full licences
- Setting standards for practice
- Dealing with concerns about whether a doctor is attaining the set standards for practice
- Running quality assurance of Medicine degrees within the UK to ensure the necessary standards are met

BMA

The **British Medical Association** is the trade union for doctors practising in the UK and it's a professional body, with roles in research and publishing.

BNF

The **British National Formulary** (BNF) is a reference resource for medical professionals to consult on the selection and use of medicines.

SMC

The **Scottish Medicines Consortium** is Scotland's equivalent of NICE (it looks at the effectiveness and value for money of new drugs).

NICE

The **National Institute for Health and Care Excellence** (NICE) is a special health authority that operates nationally in England and Wales. It was set up in 1999 to reduce the effect of the 'postcode lottery' where patients received differing levels of treatment and care from the NHS depending on where they live.

Areas in which NICE publishes guidelines are:

- Recommendations on drugs – to ensure equal access to drugs that are deemed clinically and cost effective
- Guiding healthcare – issuing guidance on effective ways to treat patients and prevent ill health
- Health promotion – guidance for public sector workers on maintaining good health

EWTD

Since 2009, the **European Working Time Directive** (EWTD) has restricted the number of hours people in the UK can work. The main measures of the EWTD are:

- The average working week must be 48 hours or less.
- There must be a daily rest of 11 hours per 24-hour period.
- There must be right to a day off each week.
- There must be right to a rest break if the working day is longer than 6 hours.

Ethics and law

We have tried to succinctly describe and explain some key concepts in the field of medical ethics and law. Some parts of the information below are beyond the level you are expected to know, but it will be impressive if you can use any of the following in your interviews (and we hope you find it interesting!).

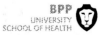

The four key principles of medical ethics

1. **Beneficence:** Doing the best you can for patients.

2. **Non-maleficence:** 'First, do no harm'.

3. **Respect for patient autonomy:** Giving competent, informed patients control over what happens to their body. This means that patients can refuse life-saving treatment. (**Note.** Autonomy = self-rule.)

4. **Justice:** Treating patients fairly. This includes fair access to treatments and fair access to our limited medical resources.

Consent

There are three components required for consent (a patient giving their doctor permission to treat / examine them / take bloods etc)

- Competence
- Non-coercion
- Information

Competence: The patient should be able to understand the information given to them, retain it long enough to weigh it up, and then be able to communicate their decision to the doctor.

Non-coercion: There should be no outside pressure/influence on the patient forcing them to make a decision that's not their own.

Information: The patient should be given all of the relevant information they need in a way they can understand.

To perform any procedure a doctor must have valid consent (patient is informed, competent and their decision is voluntary).

If someone touches another person in a harmful manner without consent they may be liable for battery (trespass to the person). The same applies to doctors: if a doctor does something without valid consent they are committing a crime (battery) and can be prosecuted.

If a patient is competent (and non-coerced) they can refuse any (including life-saving) treatment. Doctors should respect this and, if they do not, they will face prosecution.

Competence

Patients 16 years (not 18!) or older are assumed to be competent until proven otherwise. However, if a 16/17 year old refuses consent, their decision can be overridden by their parents or a court, to act in their best interests.

Competence is based solely on the patient's capacity and not the decision they make. A competent patient can refuse any treatment, even if it will lead to their death. 'Treatment' includes food and ventilation.

Competence is not universal. A patient may be competent to consent to one treatment, but not to another.

A child (under 16 years old) is presumed to lack capacity to consent to treatment. However, a child under 16 who is deemed to have capacity by their doctor can give consent.

Note. A patient can refuse treatment, but cannot demand it. Doctors do not have to follow patient demands for treatment.

Negligence

A doctor is negligent if there's a breach in duty of care **and** harm is done.

A doctor could be negligent if they do not give enough information to the patient (required for valid consent).

Patient's best interests

Incompetent adults should be treated in their best interests.

The doctor decides what's in their patient's best interests, by looking at previously expressed wishes, the patient's beliefs, and by consulting the patient's friends and relatives.

Euthanasia

Euthanasia literally means 'good death'. Generally, it's defined as the termination of a sick patient's life to relieve them of their suffering.

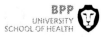

Types of euthanasia

- Voluntary vs. involuntary vs. non-voluntary

  - Voluntary: Competent request to die

  - Involuntary: Death is against a competent request to live

  - Non-voluntary: Patient is not competent to make a request

- Active vs. passive

  - Active: Action results in patient's death

  - Passive: Patient allowed to die (life-prolonging treatment withheld or withdrawn), ie an omission not an act

Assisted suicide: Patient helped to kill himself/herself (eg drugs left by bedside).

Active euthanasia ('mercy killing') is illegal in the UK, but it remains legal in some parts of the world. Passive euthanasia is legal in the UK.

Doctrine of double effect: A doctor in the UK can give pain-relieving drugs to a patient, even if the drugs hasten the patient's death, so long as the intention is to relieve pain and not to hasten death (this may be foreseen but should not be the intention). This is known as indirect euthanasia.

There are a number of arguments for and against you should be aware of …

'For' euthanasia:

- Autonomy: Everyone has the right to control what happens to their body, including when and how they die.

- Right to life includes right to die: Right to life is not just a right to exist, but also a right to a good life quality. A 'good death' is an important part of this.

- Suffering: Suffering is bad. Euthanasia relieves suffering.

- Is death a bad thing?: If death is not bad, many of the arguments against euthanasia fall apart.

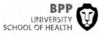

- Regulation: If euthanasia can be appropriately regulated the 'slippery slope' (see below) situation cannot occur.

- Suicide: Attempting and committing suicide is legal. Patients unable to take their own life, who competently want to die, should be helped to die.

- Resources: The limited resources of the NHS can be used by other patients.

'Against' euthanasia:

- Sanctity of life: Life is sacred (eg a gift from God).

- Slippery slope argument: Who says what 'suffering' is? If voluntary euthanasia is legalised standards will slip and involuntary euthanasia will (inevitably) occur.

- Devaluing life situations: Allowing euthanasia of the severely disabled means society does not see their life as worth living.

- Palliative care: Proper palliative care avoids the need for euthanasia.

- Vulnerable exploited: Vulnerable people may feel pressurised into dying, if they feel like a burden, or they are forced into it by friends/family or financial pressure (end-of-life care is expensive).

- Desire to die: Desire to die may be a fleeting thought, or be made in a confused state (ie when not competent).

Confidentiality

Doctors have a duty to protect their patients' confidentiality. This trust is vital for the doctor-patient relationship.

However, there are some circumstances where doctors have a legal duty to disclose patient information:

- Notifiable diseases (eg smallpox)

- Court order

- Public safety (eg HIV patients refusing to tell their partner, or warning the DVLA about an unsafe driver who refuses to stop driving)

Abortion

Abortion is the termination of pregnancy.

Abortion can be performed up to 24 weeks (before viability – when a foetus can survive outside the womb) with the woman's consent, on wide grounds. Two doctors are needed to justify the abortion.

(Abortion after 24 weeks is a minefield, and can only be allowed to prevent risk of considerable harm to either the mother or the future child.)

There are a number of arguments for and against you should be aware of.

'For' abortion (pro-choice):

- A foetus is not a person: Only people have a moral status. A foetus has no moral status, so it's not wrong to kill it.

- Bodily rights: A foetus is part of the woman's body. A woman has control over her body. A woman can choose to kill a foetus inside her body.

- Back-alley abortions: Banning abortions means women are more likely to perform unsafe abortions outwith the regulated health service.

- Rape victim: A child resulting from rape may make it impossible for women to forget that traumatic experience.

'Against' abortion (pro-life):

- A foetus is a person: It's wrong to kill an innocent human being. A foetus is a human being. It's therefore wrong to kill a foetus.

- Sanctity of life: Life is sacred (a gift from God).

- Right to life: Every living thing has a right to life.

- Help from society: Women don't need to be offered abortions; they need financial and social support to raise their children without having to compromise on their life situation.

- Adoption: Many families would love to adopt a child. There is no such thing as an unwanted child.

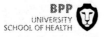

- Pregnancy is not the problem: summed up by Megan Clancy:

  'There are women who are raped and become pregnant;

  the problem is that they were raped, not that they are pregnant.

  There are women who are starving who become pregnant;

  the problem is that they are starving, not that they are pregnant.

  There are women in abusive relationships who become pregnant;

  the problem is that they are in abusive relationships, not that they are pregnant.'

Gradualist approach: There is another approach to abortion: gradualism. This involves the concept of personhood, ie when a foetus is deemed to become a 'person'. The gradualist position takes the stance that the foetus gains in moral status as pregnancy progresses.

Doctors who have a conscientious objection to abortion or to a particular patient having an abortion have to refer patients on to other doctors.

Advance Directives

Advance Directives are made at a time when a person is competent and they state what they want to happen to them if they are ill and incompetent. They can give preferences, spell out what they want to happen in certain situations or give a friend/relative their decision-making power ('proxy directive').

Medical conditions and disease processes

We have compiled a list of some key medical conditions and disease processes you should know about. You will come across many of these during your work experience placements and may indeed know a friend or relative who has suffered from or currently suffers from one of these. They also appear frequently in the news, so you should have a good basic understanding about them. You could be asked about these during an interview, especially if you have mentioned them in your Personal Statement or you bring it up during interview.

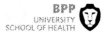

Asthma

- Breathlessness is induced by bronchoconstriction, which is narrowing of the lung's main tubes (the bronchi). The bronchi can fill with mucus making breathing difficult in an asthma attack.

- Asthma is common, affecting one in five households in the UK. There are triggers, such as animals or pollen, which can cause an asthma attack.

- Asthma can cause breathlessness, wheezing and coughing. Exercise often leads to these symptoms, and inhalers may be required. Asthmatics often have worse symptoms early in the morning.

- Asthma is diagnosed by taking a history and by performing a lung function test.

- Respite commonly comes in the form of salbutamol found in blue inhalers. Brown steroid inhalers can also be used. Patients will be advised to avoid their asthma attack triggers.

Atherosclerosis

- This is a disease process that involves the accumulation of fatty deposits (atheroma), which causes narrowing of arteries, as atheromatous plaques form and implant in the tissue lining the vessels.

- Cholesterol plays a major role in the build-up of these plaques, which can break off, leading to occlusion (blockage) of arteries, causing ischaemia (lack of blood supply and hence oxygen and energy) and infarction (heart attack or stroke).

Cancer

- Cancer is uncontrolled and abnormal cell growth. Cancer can be benign or malignant.

- Benign means that the cancer growth will not spread, remaining contained at its site of origin. Malignant tumours, however, invade surrounding tissues, and metastasise (move) to other parts of the body, to form a secondary tumour (with the initial tumour being called the primary).

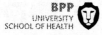

- Genetics, lifestyle choices (eg smoking and lung cancer) and infections (eg HPV and cervical cancer) can all play a part in the development of cancer.

- Symptoms include tiredness, cachexia (severe weight loss) and pain.

- Diagnosis is by imaging and histology (looking at the cells under a microscope).

- Treatment includes chemotherapy, radiotherapy and/or surgery to kill/remove cancerous cells. All of the treatments have serious side effects, and cancer can return at a later date, especially if not all is killed at the time.

COPD

- COPD is Chronic Obstructive Pulmonary Disease and involves a collection of lung conditions including emphysema and chronic bronchitis. Emphysema occurs when there's a loss of the elasticity of the lungs (in the alveolar air sacs). Bronchitis is inflammation and infection of the bronchi (the lung's main tubes).

- COPD causes increased mucus, inflamed airways and scarring, leading to narrowed airways. This makes breathing difficult, and patients get a (phlegm-producing) cough.

- The main cause of COPD is smoking, which damages and scars the airways over time.

- Diagnosis is by history taking and lung function tests.

- The best thing for a COPD patient to do is to stop smoking. Medications like inhalers can help, and surgery is possible for a small number of patients.

Dementia

- Dementia is generally a disease of old age. Alzheimer's disease ('plaques' and 'tangles' lead to death of brain cells) is the most common cause of dementia. Strokes can also cause dementia.

- Patients become forgetful and struggle with day-to-day activities. Personality changes occur at end-stage dementia.

- Diagnosis is by history taking (from the patient and their carers) and brain imaging (CT, PET, SPECT or MRI scans).

- Dementia has no cure and is progressive but not fatal; patients generally die from other causes after about a decade with dementia.

Diabetes

- There are two types of diabetes: Type 1, or early-onset, is a failure of the pancreas to produce enough insulin. Type 2 involves the loss of sensitivity to insulin by body cells. Type 2 is more common for adults and is generally because of obesity or lack of exercise.

- With type 1 there are the 'typical' symptoms of polydipsia (thirst), polyuria (frequent urination) and weight loss. Type 2 is often asymptomatic (no symptoms present).

- Diagnosis is by taking a history and by taking blood sugar readings.

- Type 1 is treated using insulin injections (to make up for shortage) whereas type 2 is treated with lifestyle changes (weight loss, dieting and more exercise). If this fails, a number of drugs can be tried. Insulin injections are an option if all else fails.

Heart attack

- Medically known as a myocardial infarction (MI), a heart attack occurs when a coronary artery supplying the heart with oxygen is occluded (blocked). This leads to a lack of oxygen (ischaemia) to the muscle, which leads to death of the heart tissue (infarction).

- MIs are diagnosed by taking a full history of the patient and by performing an ECG (recording the electrical activity of the heart, which is interrupted by dead tissue, giving a tell-tale trace). Another test analyses the blood for troponin, an enzyme released from dying heart cells.

- Heart attacks are treated using thrombolytic (clot-busting) drugs such as streptokinase, or by coronary angioplasty (a balloon is pumped up inside the blocked artery inside a mesh stent, which keeps the vessel open).

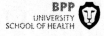

Heart disease

- Coronary Heart Disease (CHD) is the biggest killer in the UK. Also known as ischaemic heart disease, CHD occurs when the blood supply to the heart muscle is interrupted or blocked by fatty plaques (atherosclerosis) in the coronary arteries. CHD can cause angina (chest pain), lead to a heart attack (MI) or cause heart failure (when the heart becomes too weak to pump blood around the body).

- Diagnosis is made by risk assessing the patient, by looking at family history, lifestyle factors and their medical history. Blood samples are also taken. Diagnosis may be confirmed by ECG, MRI, CT or by coronary angiography.

- The best thing for a high-risk patient to do is to work on achieving and maintaining a healthy lifestyle (regular exercise, healthy eating, stopping smoking etc). Pharmacological interventions are possible (eg statins to lower blood cholesterol), as well as surgery.

High cholesterol

- High cholesterol is technically known as hyperlipidaemia or hypercholesterolaemia (= high; cholesterol; of the blood).

- Cholesterol is an important part of the diet, but too much (of the 'bad' kind, see below) is dangerous.

- Cholesterol can be split into two 'types': LDL and HDL. LDL, low-density lipoprotein ('bad cholesterol'), takes cholesterol from the liver to cells, and excess cholesterol builds up in artery walls (atherosclerosis). HDL ('good cholesterol') returns excess and cellular cholesterol to the liver where it is broken down or removed as waste.

- An unhealthy diet, smoking, diabetes and hypertension all make cardiovascular (heart attack) and cerebrovascular (stroke) problems more likely with high cholesterol levels.

- Statins are used to control high cholesterol.

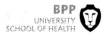

Hypertension

- Hypertension is high blood pressure, and is classed as above 140/90 mmHg for a number of weeks (systolic – heart pumping / diastolic – heart at rest).

- Hypertension is often asymptomatic (there are no symptoms), which is why regular blood pressure tests are important in adulthood.

- There are several risk factors for hypertension, the main ones being: increased body mass index (see obesity section below), family history, high salt/alcohol/caffeine intake, and stress.

- The best ways to lower blood pressure are actions targeting these modifiable risk factors. Therefore patients at risk should eat healthily, lower their alcohol consumption, take time to have a 'breather' to relieve stress, exercise more, and reduce caffeine and salt intake. Alongside lifestyle changes, medications can be given (antihypertensive drugs).

Obesity

- The body mass index (BMI) system is used to classify people as overweight/obese (and also as underweight). BMI is calculated as weight (kg) divided by height (m) squared, ie kg/m^2. A BMI from 25 to 29 is classed as overweight. Above 30 is classed as obesity ('morbid' obesity above 40).

- Obesity is often due to lifestyle choices: people who eat too much and exercise too little. However, there are some medical reasons for obesity.

- Obesity can lead to hypertension. Obesity is a key risk factor for developing a number of conditions. These include: stroke, type 2 diabetes, heart disease, and some cancers. Obesity is very dangerous for both mother and child during pregnancy.

- A healthy diet and a good exercise regime are essential. Support from others can be effective (think about Weight Watchers or Slimming World etc). Surgery is only offered as a last resort.

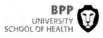

- As well as leading to dangerous conditions, obesity causes immediate problems: breathlessness, joint pain, sweating, trouble sleeping … The list is long, but it's worth remembering the patient's self-esteem. This can be a vicious circle, where obesity creates low self-esteem, leading to comfort eating.

Stroke

- There are two types of stroke: haemorrhagic and ischaemic. Haemorrhagic stroke occurs when a blood vessel bursts, leading to blood leakage into the brain itself. Ischaemic stroke occurs when a clot blocks a blood vessel supplying the brain.

- Diagnosis is by taking a full history and brain imaging (CT or MRI scan).

- It's worth remembering the mnemonic FAST: Face (can't raise both corners of mouth to smile), Arms (can't raise both arms), Speech (speech becomes slurred) and Time (which means call 999 fast!).

- The two types are managed differently. Haemorrhagic strokes are treated with antihypertensive drugs to maintain a safe blood pressure, and anticoagulant therapy is reversed. Surgery may be performed. Ischaemic strokes are treated initially with clot-busting (thrombolytic) drugs, then with anticoagulants (eg warfarin) and aspirin (to thin the blood). The clot can also be mechanically removed.

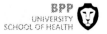

Chapter 4

Questions and answers

Motivation and understanding

1. Why do you want to study Medicine?

2. Was there anything or anyone that inspired you to do Medicine?

3. Why this Medical School?

4. What do you know about the way Medicine is taught here?

5. What do you know of PBL? Is it a good way to learn?

6. What are the differences between a doctor and a nurse? Why don't you want to be a nurse?

7. What would you do if you don't get a place this year?

8. Can you tell us about any particular life experiences that you think may help you in a career in Medicine?

9. What area of Medicine would you like to specialise in?

10. What impact do you hope to make in the field of Medicine?

11. What do you think the job of being a doctor entails, other than treating patients?

12. What makes a good doctor?

13. How would you contribute to this university?

14. Why do some people drop out of Medical School?

15. What are the downsides of Medicine?

16. What do you look forward to the most when you think about becoming a doctor?

17. How would you want your patients to describe you?

18. What steps have you taken to try to find out whether you really do want to become a doctor?

19. Take us through your Personal Statement.

20. Why do you believe you have the ability to undertake the study and work involved?

21. Is there anything you would change at this Medical School?

1. **Why do you want to study Medicine?**

   This is one of the hardest questions to answer. Some people might not have a definitive reason; some people might have hundreds of reasons. The main thing is to be honest; there's no point making something up and then being caught out when the interviewers delve deeper.

   - Rule of three

   - Use an anecdote

   - Ensure you answer the question: why Medicine specifically (as opposed to nursing, physiotherapy etc)?

   'The initial experience that got me interested in becoming a doctor was when I was diagnosed with Wolff-Parkinson-White syndrome. It was my first real involvement with hospitals, healthcare professionals and Medicine. I will always remember my astonishment at how calm all the doctors were even in my most serious episodes. Yet they were all caring, making me feel comfortable and reassuring me that I was going to be fine. That experience gave me the platform to build up my interest in Medicine.

   My interests and personality also drew me to the profession. My fascination with how the human body works, coupled with the fact I've always enjoyed helping people in any way I can, makes me believe Medicine is the right path for me. Becoming a doctor would allow me to help people as well as develop my knowledge of the workings of the human body.

   It was my work experience that reassured me that Medicine is the right choice. In all my placements I was in awe at how caring and compassionate all the doctors were and how they always made sure all their actions were done in the patients' best interests. After seeing the teamwork and dedication needed, I knew I would enjoy working in this capacity. It was an experience at my most recent placement that made me know for certain that I want to become a doctor. There was a woman with cancer in her breast and the only course of action was a mastectomy. Fortunately the surgeon I was shadowing was able to perform a breast reconstruction. The thing that got to me wasn't how good the reconstruction was; it was the patient's reaction. I remember her crying and saying she felt he had saved her life twice as she didn't think she could have coped with only one breast. It was then that I knew that if I have the opportunity to help people in this way that I must take it.'

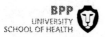

2. **Was there anything or anyone that inspired you to do Medicine?**

   This can be a difficult question to answer if there's no obvious person or event. Be honest if there is nothing you can think of, but make sure you show you're still passionate about doing Medicine. This answer should also be found in your response to 'Why Medicine?'

   - The key thing is to be truthful. Interviewers will know if you're making it up.

   - Ideas: a personal experience; an occasion in your work experience; an inspirational person in your life.

   - Uphold confidentiality.

   > 'During my work experience at a breast cancer clinic I met a patient who had a tumour in her right breast. Unfortunately, the only option was a mastectomy. The surgeon was able to perform a breast reconstruction. What got to me wasn't how good the reconstruction was; it was the patient's reaction. I remember her crying and saying she felt the surgeon had saved her life twice as she didn't think she would have been able to cope mentally with just one breast. This had a profound impact on me. I realised if I have the opportunity to change someone's life like this, I must take it.'

3. **Why this Medical School?**

   The interview panel is checking whether you actually want to come to their Medical School. Show them you've researched the surrounding area and the Medical School; read the prospectus and visit the website. Also include why this particular Medical School is suited to you. Remember there are hundreds of people trying to get into every Medical School so make sure you are fully motivated to go to all of your choices.

   - Talk about the city, the university and the course

   - Bring in what you've learnt from talking to staff and students during Open Days

   - Be passionate

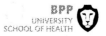

'I have lived in Manchester for almost all my life. It is a fantastic city to grow up in; there's so much to do, but I feel there's so much more to explore. Coming to Manchester will give me a different insight into life in this great city. However, the biggest attraction for me is the course. I believe the PBL course would suit me perfectly. I've always enjoyed working in teams. In my opinion working in a group to solve challenges as well as being encouraged to research topics on my own will develop important attributes needed as a doctor such as teamwork, communication skills and self-motivation. Not forgetting the clinical exposure and early patient contact, which makes Manchester stand out. These early experiences will give me the opportunity to further develop my people skills.

I have also talked extensively with students at the university, about the course and the university itself. They've all been unanimous in their praise for the university. They have said the course is demanding, but told me that with my work ethic and personality I will enjoy overcoming the challenges I will face on the course. I can really see myself enjoying studying Medicine here.'

4. **What do you know about the way Medicine is taught here?**

   The interviewers will be checking that you're interested enough to research the way you will be taught at their university. It's vital that you can give an articulate response and show that your research has let you make an informed choice. You should make it clear why their curriculum and course structure appeals to you.

   - Research the course beforehand – using the university website, their prospectus and by speaking to current medical students on Open Days.

   - Medical Schools differ in their way of teaching.

   - Include information such as: style of teaching, patient contact, dissection or prosection, Student Selected Components/ Modules/Activities, placements available, and elective and intercalation opportunities.

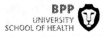

> *'I am really interested in the way Medicine is taught at Birmingham. I feel the integrated approach would suit my style of learning well. Being taught the foundations of basic medical science through lectures and tutorials in addition to practical clinical work and early patient contact during GP placements will all help me learn the various skills needed as a doctor. The first two years are spent learning about the human body via a systems-based approach. We will also learn about the psychology and sociology of health and illness as well as medical ethics. The third year is spent developing our clinical skills and learning more about patient management whilst spending time with patients in clinics. In the final two years we continue to hone our clinical skills through varied placements in primary and secondary care. I'm really looking forward to the Student Selected Activities that are available here. One of the students I spoke to on the Open Day said she undertook a fascinating project and was able to present her work afterwards at a conference. These SSAs will give me the chance to further explore areas of interest. The opportunity to carry out an elective is another appeal. All of these factors make Birmingham a great place to study Medicine.'*

5. **What do you know of PBL? Is it a good way to learn?**

    Problem-based learning (PBL) is a method used at many universities (see page 123 for further information). It is worth reading up about it even if you don't apply to a university that employs PBL primarily, as they might ask you to compare their style of teaching to PBL. If you are applying to a PBL university, make sure to include why PBL is suited to you.

    - Don't panic if you don't know every single detail of PBL.
    - Include what it involves and what the main features are.
    - Don't be fooled by leading questions. Give both sides.

'Problem-based learning involves a group of students working on a case study. After an initial meeting to discuss current understanding and what the key learning outcomes are, students go away and read around the subject matter. They then come back and discuss their findings and come up with a plan of action.

On the one hand, PBL improves vital qualities needed as a doctor such as communication and problem-solving skills, teamwork and self-directed learning. However, a possible flaw in PBL is that students won't know the depth they have to research to, so they might research too superficially or focus on details that are not very relevant. This can have an adverse effect on their learning. However, I feel the positives outweigh the negatives, as through experience students will learn how much they have to understand. There is also the issue that some students may not pull their weight in the group but dealing with this will improve management skills and enable us to become effective doctors.'

6. **What are the differences between a doctor and a nurse? Why don't you want to be a nurse?**

   This is a difficult question. The worst thing to do is to disregard the nursing profession. Make sure you know the different roles and duties of both a doctor and a nurse so you can show why being a doctor is better suited to you.

   • Most importantly, recognise the importance of nurses and the need for teamwork in a multidisciplinary healthcare team

   • Explain the differences between nurses and doctors

   • Tell of your passion to become a doctor and the reasons why

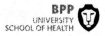

> 'Each member of the healthcare team performs a specialised role in the care of a patient. It is important to recognise this and for professionals to complement each other in their work. Doctors are the ones that examine, diagnose and manage the treatment plan, whilst nurses care for the patient and administer the treatment. I've seen first-hand the amazing work nurses do and I personally feel they deserve more credit. It could be said that nurses provide a higher proportion of the one-to-one care. Both doctors and nurses have to be leaders, teachers, good at managing people and able to make tough decisions. They both face new and difficult challenges every day. However, it is the role and qualities required of a doctor that appeals to me – as the person with ultimate responsibility for their patients. Doctors lead their multidisciplinary team. Another reason why I want to be a doctor is the training given - I'm very excited about learning about the human body in health and illness in detail. Shadowing doctors during work experience, and seeing the work that they do and the skills they possess, made me determined to follow this path.'

7. **What would you do if you don't get a place this year?**

   Unfortunately this is a real possibility. However, the interviewer is more interested in how you deal with setbacks. So show them you're mature enough to think about the possibility of it happening and that you have an idea of what you're going to do.

   • They're checking how passionate you are to become a doctor, even if a major setback occurs.

   • Options are: take a gap year, apply abroad or apply for something else such as an allied healthcare profession and reapply for Medicine.

   • Show that you've thought of all the possibilities but your passion to do Medicine wins through.

'I've considered the possibility because I realise how competitive it is to get into Medical School. Not getting a place would be hugely disappointing. However, this would not stop me from fulfilling my dream. I would take a year out and strengthen my application by gaining further work experience, so I leave Medical Schools with no option but to give me a place. I believe a gap year would also enable me to improve my communication and management skills through the voluntary and paid work I will be doing, which will be beneficial for the future. I would not give up and I can't see myself doing anything other than Medicine.'

8. **Can you tell us about any particular life experiences that you think may help you in a career in Medicine?**

    There is no point making something up and then being caught out. Talking about an experience you had during your work shadowing, or if you have been a patient and experienced patient-centred Medicine first-hand, is a great idea.

    *   Be honest
    *   Try to give an example
    *   Make it personal

    'Having spent a lot of time in hospital due to my Wolff-Parkinson-White syndrome, I have had a lot of contact with doctors. I can use this experience of being the patient to know what patients look for in their doctor: a calm and collected nature, reassurance, care and compassion. I could also see myself taking on the duties required of a doctor such as the ability to make complex decisions and help lead a wider team in the care of patients.'

9. **What area of Medicine would you like to specialise in?**

    It can be hard thinking this far ahead, especially with so little experience and exposure to clinical Medicine. There's no pressure in deciding right there and then what you want to do when you're a doctor. The interviewers just want to know if there are any areas of Medicine that interest you and why. Also, make clear that you understand that you'll come across a range of areas of Medicine that might interest you during your learning.

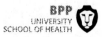

- Show you have thought of areas of Medicine you're interested in

- Refer to work experience and wider reading

- Be open to the idea that you might find something you enjoy more during your training

'I've always enjoyed working with children. This was further reinforced by my work experience on a paediatric ward, so Paediatrics appeals to me. However, it is a long journey to become a doctor so I might find another area of Medicine that attracts me. It would be foolish to set my mind on just Paediatrics at this stage, so I'm going to go into Medical School with an open mind and make the most of all the experiences available.'

10. What impact do you hope to make in the field of Medicine?

This is a great opportunity to share your ambitions and goals. However, make sure they are reasonable and achievable. It is okay if you have no set goals for your career; be honest and tell the interviewers what you would enjoy doing rather than making something up.

- Show interviewers you've thought about your future and have goals you want to accomplish

- Try to show a bit of humility

- Have realistic goals

'Personally I feel the greatest impact I can have is with the patients I treat. If all my patients are happy with the care they receive and know I have helped them to the best of my ability, then I will have accomplished my main goal. I believe a key part of being a doctor is to pass on knowledge and experience to younger doctors and I look forward to being able to teach the next generation. Another key role of doctors is to be an active part of the wider scientific community, contributing to research and improving the care I give to patients based on this.'

11. What do you think the job of being a doctor entails, other than treating patients?

Your work experience will give you an understanding of what doctors do. Doctors do not just treat patients; there are other important roles that doctors must fulfil.

- Draw upon and refer to your work experience

- They're making sure you know the roles doctors have

- Include things such as: reassuring patients, working with other doctors, leading the multidisciplinary team, attending meetings, teaching younger doctors and students, research, journalism etc

> *'My work experience gave me an insight into the various roles a doctor has to fulfil. They have to: talk to patients, comfort them, reassure them and make sure they know what the medical team are planning to do. They work alongside other doctors, nurses and allied members of the multidisciplinary team to decide on the best ways to treat and manage patients. Another significant role is teaching younger doctors and medical students – passing on their knowledge and experience. I can't wait to take part in all of these roles.'*

12. What makes a good doctor?

The interviewers want to make sure you know what patients want from their doctors. This is something you will have gathered during your work experience; you can see compassion, confidence and the way they interact with others, and how this puts patients at ease.

- They want to know what you think the important qualities of a doctor are

- Think back to your work experience and the doctors you shadowed there

- Try to include qualities you think you have in yourself

You can split the qualities into personal (compassion, empathy etc) and professional (teamwork, leadership, interpersonal) ones.

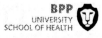
BPP
UNIVERSITY
SCHOOL OF HEALTH

'Integrity is of utmost importance.

Doctors must be caring and compassionate so they can empathise with their patients. Without this, patients won't feel comfortable with the doctor, which will affect the doctor-patient relationship and how well the patient can be treated.

Being a leader and a great team player is a must for good doctors; they not only have to lead and manage teams but they have to make sure they can effectively work with a variety of different people in the multidisciplinary healthcare team.

A good doctor must always be looking to better themselves so they can always provide the best care for patients. Lifelong learning is essential.

Finally, they must be good communicators, as they have to relay information to patients and other colleagues so they can understand what is happening. I think I have displayed all of these qualities in different situations, and I look forward to honing these during Medical School and beyond.'

13. **How would you contribute to this university?**

You can include ideas such as: your work ethic and your involvement in societies and clubs.

- Say how hard you work and how dedicated you will be to the course

- Mention activities that you do currently and ones that you might want to take up whilst at university

- Talk about your skills as a leader and as a team player

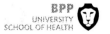

> *'I believe I would bring many things to this university. Firstly, my attitude: I am always willing to learn and work. I am enthusiastic in everything I do, always giving 100%. I'm also the sort of person who looks to help others out whenever I can.*
>
> *I have had a lot of experience in organising and taking part in societies so I would be looking to join one and take responsibility for the society's success when I can.*
>
> *Finally, I'm a keen sportsman playing football for a local team and basketball for my school, captaining both teams. I hope I can get involved with the sports teams here and if possible represent the university.*
>
> *I feel I have a lot to offer to this university, and can't wait to get involved in student life here.'*

14. Why do some people drop out of Medical School?

You have to show that you understand that Medicine is a demanding course.

- Ideas to include: high workload, stress, patients dying, long hours, the course length

- Be modest, you haven't faced those situations yet so you don't how you will cope

- Try to include the qualities you have that might be able to deal with those problems and show the passion that will keep you going

> *'Medical School is really tough. I've spoken to current students and doctors who've been through it so I'm not naïve to the challenges ahead. I think the biggest factor would be the enormous workload students have to face. The workload is a daunting prospect, but I hope my ability to break tasks into manageable chunks will stop me from becoming overwhelmed. Another issue that might cause people to drop out will be coping with patients dying. I have been lucky to not have to deal with that personally, but I'm hoping I will be able to develop some emotional resilience to not let a patient's death affect my ability to treat other patients. I'm positive Medicine is the right career for me, and this will motivate me to get through whatever challenges I face.'*

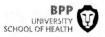
BPP
UNIVERSITY
SCHOOL OF HEALTH

15. What are the downsides of Medicine?

This is not a trick question; every job has downsides. The key is to show how you'll be able to deal with the setbacks you will face.

Alternatively, you could be asked: How would you dissuade someone from going into Medicine? Drawbacks include: high workload, stress, long hours, many years in training, patients dying, an inability to 'help' some patients, and the unfashionable aspects of the job.

- Outline the main downsides
- Say how you'll overcome them
- Understand you might have to ask for help from others

'In my opinion the two biggest setbacks in Medicine are the stress caused by the high workload and dealing with patients dying. Being a doctor is going to be very stressful at times, so I will find ways to relax. Reading, playing sport and going out with friends all help. However, I find the best way for me to cope with the workload is to put things into perspective so I don't get overwhelmed.

Dealing with patients dying is going to be a new experience for me. I think in that situation I would review the case ensuring I am happy with everything I did. I might consult senior doctors and see if they would have done anything differently. However, I know there is no easy way to deal with losing a patient. I would have to be able to develop an emotional resilience so I would still be able to carry on treating other patients but being wary not to lose my caring nature.'

16. What do you look forward to the most when you think about becoming a doctor?

This will be individual to you. Make sure you give an honest answer and show enthusiasm!

- Include the things that attract you most to being a doctor

- Be passionate when you talk

- Ideas to include: new challenges every day, chance to help people, working in a team

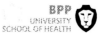

'There are so many things that I look forward to. I love the prospect of being able to help a variety of people who come to me needing help. The teamwork in a hospital is also a big attraction, there's always someone to work with or talk to when trying to help a patient. I think the thing I'm looking forward to most is the variety; no two patients are the same so there will always be new challenges. I can't wait to be part of this!'

17. **How would you want your patients to describe you?**

    Think back to your work experience and your own experiences of doctors; what are good doctors like? What would you strive to be like as a doctor?

    • Care and compassion

    • 'People skills' (leader/manager, effective communicator, team player)

    • Make patients feel comfortable (through confidence, ability and knowledge, and empathy)

    'I would want my patients to see me as a confident person; someone they can put their faith in to help them get better. I would also want them to see me as a caring person, listening to their problems and being able to empathise with them. Finally, I would want them to say I'm determined, not letting any setbacks stop me from finding a way to help them.'

18. **What steps have you taken to try to find out whether you really do want to become a doctor?**

    The interview panel is making sure you've thoroughly researched the profession and that you're passionate to learn about becoming a doctor.

    • Ideas to include: work experience, talking to doctors, reading books

    • Be honest; they might probe further about the books or articles you have read

    • Conclude with what you learnt from them and how it will make you a better doctor

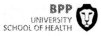

'When I first started to think about Medicine as a career, I decided to read up about Medicine. "The Rise and Fall of Modern Medicine" was a fascinating book about the development of Medicine throughout the years. "Trust Me I'm a Junior Doctor" was a humorous book that showed me the trials and tribulations I would face as I leave Medical School. Wanting to learn and understand more about Medicine, I undertook work experience both on a Paediatric Ward and on an Oncology Ward. They were both fantastic experiences for me as I saw how a hospital runs and the variety of jobs doctors must do. I also spent my time there talking to doctors, junior and senior, about their experiences. The key message was that the journey to become a doctor is a long and arduous one, but Medicine is a rewarding career. All my research and work experience reassured me that Medicine was the right path for me.'

19. Take us through your Personal Statement.

They are testing your knowledge on your application. So make sure you re-read your Personal Statement plenty of times beforehand.

- Make sure you know the key features of your Personal Statement

- Don't regurgitate; use this opportunity to emphasise the things you really wanted to highlight but might not have had the space to

- Add on the things that are unique to you; this will make you more memorable

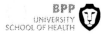

> *'I started off my Personal Statement talking about my Wolff-Parkinson-White Syndrome, as that experience gave me the platform to build up my interest in Medicine. This was because the level of care shown by the people that treated me was astounding and I felt I would enjoy doing the same thing. My school life was also a big part of my Personal Statement as it played a pivotal role in my choice to apply for Medicine. It was at school where I developed a fascination with the way the human body worked. School also gave me the opportunity to play in sports teams improving my team-working skills. I was also lucky enough to captain our team as well as become Deputy Head Boy of the school. These roles gave me a lot of responsibility, which I found tough at first but thoroughly enjoyed having and I feel they helped me become a much better leader. My work experience placements confirmed Medicine is the career for me. All of the people I met and talked to during my placements had an effect on me and helped me realise I would enjoy being a doctor.'*

20. **Why do you believe you have the ability to undertake the study and work involved?**

    This is a difficult question, so don't just rush into the answer. Take your time and think why you are suited to becoming a doctor. You could include self-directed learning examples (such as EPQ) here, as this style of learning is important in Medical School and beyond.

    - A key thing to include is your personal attributes that allow you to cope
    - Give examples of times when you have shown these attributes
    - Relate your skills to those of a doctor

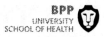

> *'I feel I have many attributes that will allow me to undertake the work involved. Firstly, my attitude. I am always willing to learn and work. This, along with my determination, makes me confident I will be able to cope with the work involved. I am also very organised and good at task management. Using these skills will mean I don't become overwhelmed when dealing with the challenges I will face. I was able to use these abilities in my final year of school when I had to juggle my deputy head duties, organising the prom, and my schoolwork. I felt I was able to accomplish each of them without compromising on my high standards. So hopefully this puts me in good stead to cope with the workload ahead.'*

21. Is there anything you would change at this Medical School?

This is a hard question to answer. The obvious answer is 'No' but you need to explain why. Another option is to say no, but tell them of something that you didn't like at first, but now do. If you do go with yes, make sure it is a minor thing that can be easily changed or you might change your mind about.

> *'No, there is not. At first I was a bit disappointed to learn dissections aren't done here. However, after reading up on what prosections are and speaking to current students, my mind changed. We are here to learn and I would be worried about damaging the body part we are studying and ruining our chance of learning from it. So I am happy with a professional helping us in our learning by doing the actual dissection.'*

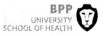

Personality

1. Tell us about yourself.

2. I see you deal with customers at work – how have you dealt with angry customers?

3. How do you cope with stress?

4. How do you think you would cope with criticism from colleagues or other healthcare professionals? / How will you cope with being criticised or even sued by patients?

5. How would you cope with patients dying?

6. What would you do if, on a night shift, you prescribed penicillin to a patient, and the patient's nurse said that you've made a mistake prescribing this?

7. Are you a leader or a follower?

8. Do you see yourself as a leader?

9. Would you say you're a great leader?

10. When have you worked in a team?

11. Do you prefer to learn alone or in groups?

12. How would you break bad news?

13. What qualities do you think other people value in you?

14. What are three positive things that one of your teachers would say about you?

15. If you had to be either a nurse or a scientist, which would you choose?

16. How would your friends describe you as a person?

17. Prove to us here and now that you are a kind person ...

    - Do you give money to beggars in the street?
    - What do you do most evenings?

18. What are your strengths and weaknesses? / Give two personal qualities you have which would make you a good doctor, and two personal shortcomings which you think you would like to overcome as you become a doctor.

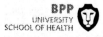

19. Do you ever get angry?

20. Tell me about a time when you have been sad or confused.

21. Is it OK for ... to have an affair?

    • Is it OK for footballers to have an affair?
    • Is it OK for a GP to have an affair with a patient?

22. What one question would you ask if you were interviewing others to study Medicine?

23. OK, so... what makes you special, and why should we give you a place at this Medical School and not someone else?

24. You are an FY1 (Junior Doctor) and your consultant turns up to work drunk. What would you do?

1. **Tell us about yourself.**

   Have a think about what this is asking of you, and why. It's important that this one doesn't throw you, and that you give a confident, well-structured response. If this is asked, it will be at the start of your interview. The first and last impressions you give to the interview panel are crucial, so make sure your response leaves a great first impression.

   A good strategy would be to start by introducing yourself. Then go on to explain your academic achievements: what courses you take and how you are doing with them. Tell them about your hobbies and interests – basically everything that makes you who you are. A good way to end would be by tying in all of the skills that you have learnt and developed, and then how these, and your work experience, led you to a career in Medicine. After all, choosing Medicine is a big part of who you are.

   - Introduce yourself
   - School and life outside of school
   - Hopes for the future

   > *'My name is … I'm 19 years old and I live in … I'm currently on a gap year; having completed my A Levels at … where I was Head Boy. I studied Chemistry, Biology, Spanish and Maths and excelled at all of them. I am an active member of the community, volunteering at … and … My gap year offers an important opportunity to experience the world of work, and I'm currently holding down several jobs to give me a good head start when it comes to paying for life at university. I enjoy cycling and reading in my spare time, and I love travelling.*
   >
   > *My compassionate nature and love of human biology led me to undertake several work experience placements in various healthcare settings. I enjoyed all of these and, alongside substantial research, decided Medicine is what I want to do for the rest of my life. I'm very passionate, highly motivated and look forward to the most rewarding of vocations.'*

2. **I see you deal with customers at work – how have you dealt with angry customers?**

   You may not have worked in a situation like this, but the question could simply be 'How do you deal with difficult people?' As a

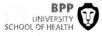

doctor, you will come across patients and their families who are angry, for whatever reason. The only way to move forward will be to explore their feelings, let them vent their anger, and then try to find a way forward together.

To do this, it's important to listen to what they have to say – you have to listen without interrupting. It's important at this stage to apologise sincerely for any shortcomings. Knowing the reason for their anger will then let you try to resolve the issue. You have to try your utmost to help, and let them know that what has happened will not occur again.

- Listen
- Apologise and be polite
- Resolve the issue

> *'During my time as a barman/waiter I've come across a huge number of personalities. Some customers have been angry. However, I feel I have the ability to diffuse these situations. I let the customers have their say, and I listen to what they are saying. I then simply say "Sorry". Although this sounds obvious, I've found it makes a huge difference. I then try to find a solution that makes the customer happy – involving management if necessary. Problems can stem from miscommunication between staff, so as a team we'd talk it through and see where the problem lies. I'd re-apologise, and assure them the mistake will not occur again.'*

3. **How do you cope with stress?**

   The actual mechanisms you use will be individual to you: be it sport, music or art etc. This question therefore overlaps with hobbies/interests, but it also delves into who you are as an individual. What keeps you focused and calm? You will have picked up strategies as you have worked through your college courses, and had to balance a heavy workload with outside interests. Coping with stress is a necessity for Medical School and life as a doctor.

   - Short-term strategies (exercise etc)
   - Long-term strategies (diet/exercise/sleep)
   - Support network

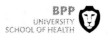

'Having already undertaken my A-Level exams, I've had to deal with stress before. During the exam period I employed various techniques to combat the rising stress levels. For example, I found that simply having a breather and counting to ten helped a lot – short breaks let you re-focus. Exercise is a great release for me too. I especially enjoy cycling, which allows me to clear my head. Above all though, I think it helps immensely to keep things in perspective, and to organise your life well – with a healthy sleep pattern and diet – which helps to keep your stress level as low as possible. Making time for friends and family is really important.'

4. **How do you think you would cope with criticism from colleagues or other healthcare professionals? / How will you cope with being criticised or even sued by patients?**

    These two questions are asking the same of you: how do you handle criticism?

    Initially, nobody likes criticism. However, there are two types of criticism: constructive and non-constructive. You should take constructive criticism on the chin, and try to resolve any of your own shortcomings. Non-constructive criticism is not helpful, and the best thing to do may be to simply let it go.

    *   Listen
    *   Acknowledge and accept
    *   Resolve issues if possible

'Although it can be very hard hearing criticism when you're trying your best for the patient, it would be a grave error of judgement to ignore these comments. I always listen to constructive criticism to try to better myself. It would be wise to not make the situation worse by arguing back if someone gives me non-constructive criticism.

With constructive criticism, I would analyse my work and see if I can relate to what they say. If I can, it would be important to try to resolve any of these issues. It may be worth thanking them for their honesty and guidance.

If being sued was a real concern after trying to resolve the problem person-to-person I would seek professional help, and hope that the patient realises how committed I am to doing the right thing.'

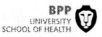
BPP
UNIVERSITY
SCHOOL OF HEALTH

5. How would you cope with patients dying?

This is something that you will find distressing as a junior doctor right through to being a consultant. The most important thing to remember is that if it affects you too much, your ability to treat other patients will be compromised. At the end of the day, the patient always comes first. To ensure this happens, you will need to have coping mechanisms to keep on going, and to maintain perspective.

One way of dealing with a patient's death would be to have a support network – people that you can talk to and reflect on what's happened with. This may be your partner, colleagues, or friends. Other healthcare professionals may be the best for this, because they face the same challenges. Another release may be sport or a creative pastime. Obviously kicking a football about or painting a picture isn't going to make everything OK but you should do whatever you feel is best for you.

- Support network (colleagues/friends/family)
- Looking after yourself (exercise/sleep/diet)
- Use patient care as the driving force to get back on track

'It would be extremely distressing, but I realise it is part of the job. I think the thing that would keep me going through these times would be my duty of care to other patients. I would remain determined to treat them to the very best of my ability. I also think it would help me to know that I'd tried my utmost to help the patient who had died.

I would share my thoughts and feelings with a colleague, who would have gone through the same and would be able to comprehend how I was feeling. I would reflect with them on what had happened, and what I had learned from it.

I would grieve privately if it were all too much, but would keep a brave face on when I'm consoling the patient's family or friends.

I think I would also make time for myself, and go cycling. I appreciate that a few hours on the bike won't make everything alright, but it would give me time to reflect on what has happened.'

6. **What would you do if, on a night shift, you prescribed penicillin to a patient, and the patient's nurse said that you've made a mistake prescribing this?**

   - Speak to the nurse and establish facts
   - Try to find a solution together
   - If you can't, speak to someone senior

   > *'It would be important to speak to the nurse, and ascertain all of the facts. Nurses have a greater continuity of care with patients, so the nurse may know something I don't. I would then try to find a way forward with the nurse. If this is impossible, and we can't come to an agreement, I would speak to somebody with more experience. Whatever happens, the patient's best interests would always be at the centre of the discussion.'*

7. **Are you a leader or a follower?**

   Don't jump the gun with this one. Are doctors always leaders? Think back to your work experience and you may remember times when the professional you were shadowing led the multidisciplinary team, but also times when they integrated themselves into the team. You should be able to do both, and let the interview panel know that you can.

   - Say you do both
   - Draw on work experience
   - Give examples where you have led and followed

   > *'I believe I have the qualities and capabilities to be both a leader and a follower. For example, as Head Boy I acted as a role model to the younger students, and as an ambassador of the school. During a school expedition, as the only Spanish speaker, I led the group through a number of challenging situations. Whilst in various committee meetings at school, I took charge and gave us direction, if needed. I've also played for numerous years in a football team, listening to the captain and coach and working with my teammates.*
   >
   > *I'd say I usually act in a following role, but when needed I can and do lead, and indeed enjoy this part of teamwork. During my work experience I saw the doctors in a dynamic balance between the two roles.'*

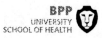

8. Do you see yourself as a leader?

You should be able to find the qualities associated with being a leader in yourself. Put these forward, but say that you can work in a team too.

- 'Yes, I do'
- Give evidence
- Acknowledge your ability to be led

> *'I believe I have the qualities of a leader instilled in me. I have brought my skills into practice on numerous occasions. For example, during my World Challenge Expedition when one of my friends fell ill I allocated jobs to each member of the team and made sure we all stayed focused. I also like working with others and letting them take charge. Sometimes I take a step back and actually lead from behind the scenes.'*

9. Would you say you're a great leader?

This is a step up from simply being a leader. You don't want to blow your own trumpet too much, but similarly you want to sell yourself. Maybe you have achievements that show your prowess – these will help to back up your answer. Maybe you've captained a sports team, led an expedition group or been in another position of responsibility.

- Sell yourself
- Use examples
- Show desire for self-improvement

> *'I definitely believe I have acquired the skills of a good leader over the past few years. My peers and teachers nominated me to act as Head Boy, which has allowed me to grow in confidence, and to develop into the leader I am today. This responsibility enhanced my leadership skills immensely, and I would like to think I'm approaching "great leader" status, if I've not already achieved it. I look forward to continuing to build upon the skills I have developed as I go through Medical School.'*

10. When have you worked in a team?

There may be several occasions when you have worked in a team. Have a think, and jot down a few of these. Maybe you were in a sports team, on a Duke of Edinburgh expedition, or were in a Young Enterprise team.

- Give examples (sport / work / committees / D of E etc)
- Skills learnt/developed
- Teamwork as a reason for wanting to do Medicine

> *'I've worked in a team on numerous occasions. I played football for several years as part of a squad, hiked in a group on my Duke of Edinburgh expedition and, on my Outlook Expedition / World Challenge expeditions, worked with others in a fundraising group and co-operated with others whilst working at the various jobs I've undertaken.*
>
> *I think team working really helps with communication and confidence.*
>
> *I have always enjoyed working in teams, and very much look forward to this aspect of Medicine.'*

11. Do you prefer to learn alone or in groups?

The best way to tackle this question is to give the pros and cons of each learning environment and then give your preferred style. You should not, however, side too heavily on either method. Both styles are found in Medicine: you will spend time learning in groups (eg in PBL and tutorials) or alone (eg in lectures, and self-directed learning).

- Pros/cons of learning alone
- Pros/cons of group work
- Arrive at a decision

> *'I think both learning styles have their merits and downfalls. Learning alone is beneficial because you know what pace is best for you, what you need extra work with and what you don't, and you may be less distracted. On the other hand, group work allows you to bounce ideas off of others, to quickly get help and assistance from like-minded students, and to share your knowledge and experience.*
>
> *Taking all things into consideration I think it depends on what I'm studying as to which style I prefer. For example, when I'm tackling a tricky diagnosis I would favour group work, because pooling knowledge would be of great benefit. However, I think I would prefer self-study when it comes to learning physiology and anatomy, because I would be able to go at my own pace.'*

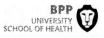

12. How would you break bad news?

Breaking bad news is part of the job. The interview panel won't expect you to be experts now, but you should be able to give a logical answer.

- Set the scene (sit down in a quiet place)
- Say that you have bad news
- Explain what has happened
- Apologise if it's your shortcoming
- See if there is anything that you can do

> *'To break bad news to ... I would first prepare them and the location. This means that I would find a quiet and safe place, sit them down, and tell them that I have bad news to tell them. This would prepare them for the shock.*
>
> *I would then explain to them what has happened, and why. I would give them some time to take in what I've said, and let them ask any questions they have. I would apologise if I had played a part in the problem, and see if there's anything I could do, or if I they want me to tell anyone else about what had happened.'*

13. What qualities do you think other people value in you?

The qualities you put forward could be: a good listener, kind, caring and selfless. These all indicate good 'people' skills, the very essence of a good doctor.

> *'Many people have said that I am a good listener. People value this because they feel comfortable sharing their thoughts and feelings with me. Lots of people respect me for my hard-working nature. I've been called selfless and mature, but I believe my kindness is the thing that others value the most.'*

14. What are three positive things that one of your teachers would say about you?

- Ability
- Attitude
- 'People skills'

> *'A teacher would probably highlight that I have the right attitude to work – I think they'd say that I'm very hard-working and self-motivated. I think they would mention my intelligence. I also believe a teacher would point out how good I am at teamwork, and how I'm able to integrate myself into different social circles.'*

15. If you had to be either a nurse or a scientist, which would you choose?

- Both are good careers
- Medicine as a mix of both
- Settle with one, explaining why

> *'Although I find both careers interesting, Medicine goes one step further and combines the two. I'm looking forward to being able to make a real difference to people in a compassionate capacity, and taking part in research, as a doctor. If I had to choose one, I think I would go with being a nurse, because as a "people person" I'm really looking forward to patient contact.'*

16. How would your friends describe you as a person?

Hopefully the characteristics they see in you match those of a good doctor.

> *'I think my friends would say that I'm a kind and caring person, a good listener and, above all, a good friend.'*

17. Prove to us here and now that you are a kind person ...

- **Do you give money to beggars in the street?**
- **What do you do most evenings?**

Questions like this can throw you, and are meant to do so. Although you will be balancing studies and a social life, it's important to make time for others. The experiences you have during voluntary placements will stick with you, and ultimately change you as a person.

- Kind with money
- Kind with time
- Attraction to Medicine

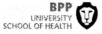

> *'I believe I am a kind person. Although I don't often give money to beggars, I have bought food and drink in the past. This way I know I really am helping. I do like to support various charities that help people in need.*
>
> *For half of the week I do voluntary work in the evening. I also give up my time during the day for various causes. I always endeavour to help people out if I can. I think my caring and compassionate nature drew me to a career in Medicine.'*

18. **What are your strengths and weaknesses? / Give two personal qualities you have which would make you a good doctor, and two personal shortcomings which you think you would like to overcome as you become a doctor.**

    It is very important to be self-aware as a doctor, and to know your own limitations. When giving your strengths back these up with an example of when you demonstrated these qualities. When you talk about your shortcomings (you will have some!) do not dress a strength up as a weakness. For example, 'I work too hard' wouldn't cut it, unless you were to say that you work really hard on projects and end up working through the night. Your weakness, in this case, would be time-management and organisation.

    - Be honest

    - Don't disguise an obvious strength as a weakness

    - Say how you are working to overcome your weaknesses and improve on your strengths

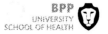

> *'I believe my main strength is my compassionate nature, which I have been able to put into practice in a number of healthcare settings. I'm a good team player, having played football from a young age, and having experienced working in groups throughout my time at secondary school. I'm able to integrate myself well into groups, which will be of great benefit when working in a multidisciplinary team.*
>
> *However, there are some things that I am going to continue to work on over the next few years, to become the best doctor I can be. I have always been quite shy on meeting people, until I get to know them and feel comfortable talking to them. However, I've been working as a barman for a few months now. My confidence is growing, and I feel much more able to approach and befriend strangers. Another thing I want to work on is my time management. I often spend vast amounts of time on projects, working well into the night, and I realise that I will have to find my own way of knowing when enough is enough with the workload at university.'*

19. Do you ever get angry?

The answer will be: Yes. You are only human; everyone gets angry at some point. However, it is how you act on that anger that is important. As a doctor, you have to be a role model to your patients (and colleagues) and be able to control your anger – with a proper outlet for your stress.

- Yes (occasionally!)
- Example situation
- Methods to calm down

> *'I do sometimes get angry, but I have ways of dealing with this anger which I think I will be able to use in my professional life. For example, I get annoyed when people are rude or ignorant, and this can turn to anger when I'm having a bad day. However, I try to keep a smile on my face, which normally helps. Having a breather and counting to ten is also a good tactic. I find that anger is more likely when you're stressed, so I try to look after myself by taking time out to exercise, and try to have a good sleep pattern.'*

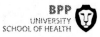
BPP
UNIVERSITY
SCHOOL OF HEALTH

20. **Tell me about a time when you have been sad or confused.**

- What made you sad/confused?

- How did you get over these feelings – who or what helped?

- Say that you can use this situation to put yourself in other people's shoes, ie you can empathise with others.

> *'I was out cycling with my Dad a few years ago and I was a few metres in front of him when I heard a sickening crash. I looked around to see my Dad on the ground, having just been hit by a car. I walked back up the road in a state of shock. My Dad put on a brave face for me and for the young driver of the car. A nurse who saw the accident happen had rushed over and helped my Dad, and she rang for an ambulance. It all happened so fast and I was sad and confused. The paramedics and the nurse comforted us all, and this kindness is something that has stuck with me. I believe that this experience opened my eyes to compassion and it allows me to empathise with people who are distressed and in need of help.'*

21. **Is it OK for ... to have an affair?**

- **Is it OK for footballers to have an affair?**
- **Is it OK for a GP to have an affair with a patient?**

This question is testing your integrity. Affairs (when someone is cheating on their partner by having the affair) are immoral. You can talk about how footballers should lead by example, as many youngsters will aspire to be like them. Doctors are pillars in the community, especially GPs. What's more, patients should feel comfortable opening up to their doctor about anything. It would be a huge breach of trust for a doctor who sees patients at their most vulnerable to then have an affair with them. This immoral behaviour could cause problems both for that doctor and for the profession as a whole.

- Affairs are wrong
- Importance of integrity for role models
- Professionalism of doctors

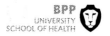

> *'Affairs are wrong, no matter who is doing the cheating. When it comes to footballers and GPs it becomes even more serious, because of the responsibility that society places on them. Footballers are role models for hundreds of thousands of children, and many follow what the footballers do, both on and off the pitch, very closely. If people see that their idol sleeps around and is unfaithful, they may be drawn to this immoral behaviour.*
>
> *GPs are pillars in the community, and should lead by example. Not only is the very act immoral, but it also sends out a worrying message with regards to sex and promiscuity, where doctors should be health advocates. Patients should feel able to talk to their GP about their most intimate problems. An affair would no doubt make this impossible, and it would be a grave breach of trust and professional conduct.'*

22. **What one question would you ask if you were interviewing others to study Medicine?**

    This is a tricky question. You don't want to say a basic or daft question but make sure you can answer it yourself. You could try to use a rare question you have practised before.

> *'I would probably ask them what makes them different from the other candidates who have applied and why they should get the place.'*

23. **OK, so … what makes you special, and why should we give you a place at this Medical School and not someone else?**

    This will almost certainly be the next question. Don't rush into the answer; it will look like it's been rehearsed. Take your time and think what would be the best way to reply.

    This may be a difficult question to answer, but remember, if you don't think you stand out, the interviewers are unlikely to either. You are unique – there may be something that you are particularly proud of which makes you special: an award, being Head Boy/Girl, a feat of endurance. Every candidate will have similar qualities: academically bright, hard-working etc. But what makes you special is everything you've seen and learnt along your journey to applying for Medicine. You will have had unique insights, been with unique patients and have a unique outlook.

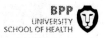
BPP
UNIVERSITY
SCHOOL OF HEALTH

> *'I believe all of my experiences to date make me special. I've met some incredible people: doctors, nurses, HCAs and patients. My desire to study Medicine has only intensified. I think one thing that makes me stand out was my appointment as Head Boy at one of the top grammar schools in the country. This responsibility allowed me to flourish personally and professionally. You should give me a place at this Medical School because I understand what it takes to be a great doctor, and I know that this Medical School is the place which will allow me to be the best I can be.'*

24. **You are an FY1 (Junior Doctor) and your consultant turns up to work drunk. What would you do?**

    Think logically and answer appropriately. Although this situation is rare, it is possible.

    - Patient safety is paramount; get the consultant away from patients

    - Ask for senior help and get other staff to cover for the consultant

    - Make sure the consultant is safe

> *'I would first ensure that the consultant is taken away from patients. This maintains patient safety and saves embarrassment for the consultant and the NHS in general. Next, I would tell someone more senior about the consultant; dealing with this situation would be beyond me as a Junior Doctor. I would ensure someone is working in the consultant's place and see to it that the consultant is safe – be it sleeping it off or sent home in a taxi. I would make sure he/she doesn't drive home!'*

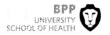

Hobbies/Interests

1. What are your hobbies?

2. What do you do in your spare time?

3. What would you do at 6:00am after a night shift in A&E to relax?

4. How do your hobbies relate to the skills needed as a doctor?

5. Which of your hobbies would you like to continue during your studies at university?

6. How do you balance work and play?

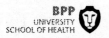

1. **What are your hobbies?**

   Being a doctor can be a very stressful job. This question is asked to see if you can show that you have a range of activities to help you relax in your future career. A good work-life balance is important.

   Many of your activities may have already been mentioned in your Personal Statement and the interviewer will want you to expand upon these.

   The key things to put across are:

   • That you are well-rounded, enjoying both solitary pursuits (eg reading, running) and team activities (playing football, playing in an orchestra)

   • Be honest

   • Explain what you gain from your hobbies

   • Explain how you would continue your hobbies whilst at university, and beyond

   > *'I enjoy several hobbies at the moment. I play football at a local club, which has greatly helped to develop my team working and communication skills, and I am keen to get involved with the MedSoc football team. I enjoy playing the guitar, which helps me to relax if I am ever feeling stressed. I have enjoyed progressing to achieve a grade 5. I also enjoy reading. I have recently finished a book called 'Medical Ethics – A Very Short Introduction' which has given me a brief insight into some of the dilemmas which medical professionals face.'*

2. **What do you do in your spare time?**

   This is similar to 'what are your hobbies?' but it is a much more open question. As with the previous question, it is important to state hobbies that can reduce stress and promote a healthy work-life balance. This question also offers an opportunity to sell yourself, as you can demonstrate the skills and personality required as a good doctor.

   Some activities you might mention are:

   • Charity/Voluntary work. This will help to show that you are a caring and compassionate person.

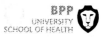

- Duke of Edinburgh Award Scheme. This will help to show your ability to work well in a team as well as your determination in completing the award.

- Medically related extra-curricular work such as an Open University course or an Extended Project. This will help to show that you have a keen interest in Medicine and can succeed in self-directed learning.

  - Sell yourself
  - Don't downplay achievements
  - Mention charity/voluntary work

> *'There are many activities which I undertake during my spare time. I have recently completed my Duke of Edinburgh Gold Award. This has required a lot of hard work, but I have enjoyed working together with the rest of my team on the hikes. I also have several hobbies such as reading and painting that I feel help me to relax if I ever feel stressed. Furthermore, I like to give back to the community through my weekly volunteering placement at a local hospice. This has helped develop my communication skills when I have been assisting patients over the past year there.'*

3. **What would you do at 6:00am after a night shift in A&E to relax?**

   As a doctor, you will find yourself in this situation and you may find that the methods you usually use to relax are impractical in this situation.

   - Think practically
   - More solitary activities
   - Why relaxation is important

> *'Being a doctor on an A&E ward can be very stressful and I understand the need for having a means of relaxing. In this situation, at 6am, there are many activities that I will be unable to do, such as playing football or a loud instrument. However, I feel that reading a book or watching a television programme can be relaxing. These activities are a good stress relief for me, and would enable me to get a good sleep, so I can give my patients the best possible care during the next shift.'*

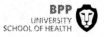
BPP
UNIVERSITY
SCHOOL OF HEALTH

4. **How do your hobbies relate to the skills needed as a doctor?**

The interviewers will want to know what you've gained from the hobbies that you do. Some traits that you may have developed that will be beneficial as a doctor include team-working skills, interpersonal communication, leadership/management skills, being a good empathiser, and self-directive learning. Listed below are why these skills are important and examples of hobbies that relate to these skills:

- **Team-working skills** – as a doctor you will be working alongside other healthcare professionals when treating a patient. It is important that you can work well with them to achieve the best patient-centred care possible.

  Examples: Playing for a football/rugby team, being part of a band, organising charity events with other people, etc

- **Communication skills** – when treating patients it is important that you can demonstrate good communication skills to effectively explore their problem. Effective communication is also important when working with your colleagues.

  Examples: Working within a team, peer mentoring, public speaking, debating societies, etc

- **Leadership and management skills** – doctors perform a leadership role within the medical team by leading the diagnosis and treatment of patients, as well as having ultimate responsibility for them.

  Examples: Being Head Boy/Girl or a Prefect, sports team captain, running a youth club, etc

- **Good empathiser** – being able to empathise with patients is essential in making a patient feel comfortable and in maintaining a good level of trust within the doctor-patient relationship.

  Examples: Voluntary work at a hospice/care home, peer mentoring, etc

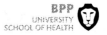

- **Self-directed learning** – being a doctor is a lifelong learning process. New treatments and medicines are being developed all the time so it is vital that a doctor is able to keep up to date with the latest advancements.

  Examples: Learning an instrument, reading medical journals, etc

- Sell yourself
- Mention a broad range of hobbies
- Why these skills are important for a doctor

> *'As a doctor there are many skills that I will require to treat my patients effectively and I believe that my hobbies have helped develop these. Firstly, playing in a football team has helped build upon my team-working skills, which will be vital when I am working in a multidisciplinary healthcare team. Secondly, my communication skills have improved during my voluntary work at my local care home, which has also enabled me to empathise better with people. Good communication is needed not only to work well with colleagues, but also to effectively interact with patients. Finally, teaching myself guitar has improved my ability to undertake self-directed learning, a skill that I will call upon often as a doctor, as studying Medicine is a lifelong learning process.'*

5. **Which of your hobbies would you like to continue during your studies at university?**

   This question gives you not only the opportunity to mention some of the extra-curricular activities that you do, but also the chance to mention what you could bring to the university. It is important, however, not to exaggerate how many activities you intend to continue whilst undertaking your Medical degree as it may seem unrealistic. Before attending the interview do some research on what clubs the university/MedSoc provides, and consider which you would be interested in when attending the university.

   - Something to relax
   - A medical society
   - Be realistic!

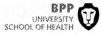
BPP
UNIVERSITY
SCHOOL OF HEALTH

'Having done some research and spoken to current medical students on the Open Day, I feel that taking part in the MedSoc football team would be ideal for me. It will give me a chance to stay active and bond with my classmates and meet students in other years. I would also like to continue being involved in charity work whilst at university, raising money for Cancer Research UK, something close to my heart. Finally, I am interested in getting involved in the anatomy society, which would also compliment my studies.'

6. **How do you balance work and play?**

Medicine is a serious commitment, but it is essential to put aside some time to relax in order to prevent yourself from becoming too stressed. This question requires you to demonstrate that you understand the importance of finding and maintaining a good work-life balance for a doctor.

'Maintaining a good balance between work and play is difficult, but essential to reduce stress and stay healthy. At the moment, I balance my studies at school with leisure activities such as reading and playing football. I find that reading a book for half an hour before I go to bed helps me to relax. I will always make time to relax when I become a doctor in order to maintain a good work-life balance and perform my best at work.'

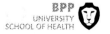

NHS / History of Medicine

1. What do you think is the most important medical advancement in the last 100 years?

2. What are the pros and cons of private healthcare?

3. What would you do if you were the Health Secretary? / How would you tackle the problems currently facing the NHS?

4. What are the implications for doctors of an ageing population?

5. Where will the NHS be in ten years' time?

6. What is the full meaning of NICE? What does NICE do?

7. What is the full meaning of GMC? What does GMC do?

8. Give an example of someone who has been struck off the GMC register.

9. How have the recent reforms changed the NHS?

10. Due to budget cutbacks there are limited resources within the NHS; what would you do to save money?

11. What's your view on the European working time directive?

12. How did the NHS start?

13. Outline what you know of postgraduate training.

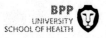

1. **What do you think is the most important medical advancement in the last 100 years?**

There have been many important medical advances in the last 100 years.

Some examples include:

- Development of **vaccines** – the last 100 years has seen the development of many successful vaccines including those against measles, mumps, rubella and diphtheria. Vaccines were also used to eradicate smallpox in the 1970s. Smallpox had previously resulted in millions of deaths per year.

- Discovery and development of **insulin** – prior to the discovery of insulin there was no known treatment for people with type 1 diabetes. In the 1920s, scientists at the University of Toronto developed extraction and purification methods for insulin. This could then be used to treat patients with diabetes via an injection. In 1977, synthetic 'human' insulin was produced in a laboratory using E. coli.

- Development of **antibiotics** – before the 20th century infections were usually treated with home remedies. The discovery of penicillin by Alexander Fleming in 1928 revolutionised the treatment of bacterial infections, and by 1945 penicillin was purified and widely available for use.

- Improved **surgical techniques** – development of anaesthetics allowed surgeons to undertake longer, more complicated operations, with far less pain for the patient. The introduction of sterilisation and antibiotics has led to a massive decline in infections caused by surgery. Research during the 20th century into blood groups has allowed surgeons to administer effective blood transfusions to patients who would otherwise have died of blood loss.

- Advances in **public health** – safe water and food inspections have helped stop millions of illnesses from developing.

- **Development of the NHS**
  - Brief overview of different advancements
  - Elaborate on the one you find most important
  - Say why it's the most important

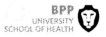

'*Over the last century there have been huge strides forward in almost every area of Medicine, from the development of vaccines to improved sanitation. In my opinion, the single most important advancement was the development of antibiotics following the discovery of penicillin in 1928 by Alexander Fleming. It has completely revolutionised treatment of bacterial diseases and has saved countless lives. Antibiotics, along with sterilisation, have also made surgery much safer by preventing infection.*'

2. **What are the pros and cons of private healthcare?**

   There are many pros and cons of private healthcare within the UK. It is important that you give a balanced view when answering this question as one of your interviewers may work for a private clinic, or even run one!

   Pros include:

   - Private healthcare helps to reduce waiting times within the NHS by treating patients who would otherwise have been on the waiting lists.

   - Private healthcare users pay towards the NHS through taxes but don't use the Service as often, allowing other NHS users to benefit more from the limited resources.

   - It helps to prevent an exodus of doctors within the UK by allowing them to supplement their wages by working in the private sector. Otherwise they may work abroad or leave Medicine.

   - It gives people the freedom to decide who treats them rather than having the Government impose that upon them.

   Cons include:

   - It exacerbates the problem of social inequality by allowing wealthier people to have access to the benefits of private healthcare that other people can't afford.

   - The private sector is financially driven and therefore the doctor may not be working in the patient's best interests. For example, unneeded investigations may be ordered by a doctor in order to claim more money off healthcare insurance.

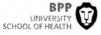

- Money spent on private healthcare could be used to improve services within the NHS that benefits everyone.

- There can be a lack of continuity of care if a patient is transferred between the NHS and private healthcare.

- If a treatment goes wrong then the patient may not always be covered to have this rectified, eg PIP breast implants. The cost of this may be placed upon the NHS.

  – Give the advantages
  – Give the disadvantages
  – Ensure you don't side too strongly one way or the other

> *'Private healthcare is available to people within the UK via healthcare insurance. There are many pros and cons with this. One advantage of private healthcare is that it helps to alleviate the problem of long waiting lists within the NHS by some patients deciding to be treated privately. Another advantage is that it provides a person with the liberty to choose whether to opt for treatment within the NHS or have it done privately. However, a disadvantage with private healthcare is that it's only available to wealthy people and therefore exacerbates the problem of social inequality. Furthermore, it is financially driven so a doctor may not work in the patient's best interests; they might over-treat the patient to get more money. Overall, I would argue private healthcare is good for the NHS. This is because it helps take the burden of patients off the NHS waiting list, whilst people who have healthcare insurance still contribute to the NHS via their taxes.'*

3. **What would you do if you were the Health Secretary? How would you tackle the problems currently facing the NHS?**

   When answering this question it is important to remember that the NHS has a finite amount of resources. Therefore, you could not simply answer this question by saying to hire more doctors/nurses, or open more hospitals. It is important to look at the big problems that the NHS faces, and offer practical solutions to them.

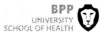

Here are two of the main challenges facing the NHS, and possible solutions.

Health

- **Issue**: Unhealthy population – lifestyle choices that people make have a big impact upon the NHS. Binge drinking, smoking and unhealthy eating cause many of the diseases that the NHS has to treat and uses up a lot of its resources.

- **Solution**: Education – prevention is better than cure. If more resources are put into educating people about the dangers of certain lifestyle choices, then less people will engage in them. This will save the NHS a lot of money that would have been spent treating preventable diseases.

Ageing

- **Issue**: Ageing population – with an ageing population there is a big increase in demand from elderly patients and diseases that are associated with them. This includes longer stays in hospital, often with multiple medication regimes (polypharmacy).

- **Solution**: More research – it is important to put more resources into developing better and more efficient treatments for diseases associated with old age. This is so they can be given the best treatment possible whilst not overspending.
  - Be realistic
  - Discuss issues
  - Give practical solutions

> *'There are many challenges facing the NHS at the moment. If I were the Health Secretary, I would put more money towards education on unhealthy lifestyles to save the NHS resources spent treating preventable diseases. I would also put more resources towards the problems of an ageing population, investing more in research into better and more efficient treatments for diseases associated with old age.'*

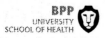
BPP
UNIVERSITY
SCHOOL OF HEALTH

4. **What are the implications for doctors of an ageing population?**

    One of the main challenges facing the NHS in the future will be the problems associated with an ageing population. The two main implications that should be considered when answering this question are:

    •   Higher expenditure within the NHS to treat a growing number of elderly patients. This means there would have to be an increase in income through taxes or a cut in spending in other areas of healthcare.

    •   More emphasis on treating patients with diseases linked to old age, such as coronary heart disease. There would also need to be more research into these diseases.

        –   More patients and a greater number of health needs
        –   An emphasis on diseases associated with old age
        –   Shift in resources needed or extra funding

    > *'A major challenge the NHS will have to adapt to in the near future is that of an ageing population. Elderly people will make up a larger proportion of the population and as they tend to have more frequent health problems this will increase the strain on the NHS. Another implication for doctors will be having more emphasis on treating diseases, such as coronary heart disease, associated with old age and focusing research on these diseases. Furthermore, there would need to either be additional funding or a shift in resources to deal with the additional problems faced.'*

5. **Where will the NHS be in ten years' time?**

    This question is concerned with the measures that will be needed to contend with the issues of the near future, such as rising obesity levels and an ageing population.

    •   Prevention over cure
    •   Changing demographics (ageing and rising obesity)
    •   New treatments

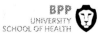

'I feel there'll be an increased focus on finding ways to prevent diseases rather than just treating them, as this saves a lot of money in the long run. Also, the NHS will have to treat more patients with diseases associated with obesity and old age. The consequences of this are that certain areas of treatment and research for those diseases will have to have their funding increased, which may have to come at the expense of other areas if funding overall does not increase. Finally, the NHS will have new treatments and techniques to treat patients in a decade's time, as Medicine is a constantly developing field.'

6. What is the full meaning of NICE? What does NICE do?

'NICE stands for the "National Institute for Health and Care Excellence". NICE is a special health authority that operates nationally in England and Wales. It was set up in 1999 to reduce the effect of the "postcode lottery" where patients received differing levels of treatment and care from the NHS based on where they live.

Areas in which NICE publishes guidelines are:

- *Recommendations on drugs – to ensure equal access to drugs that are deemed clinically and cost effective*

- *Guiding healthcare – issuing guidance on effective ways to treat patients and prevent ill health*

- *Health promotion – guidance for public sector workers on maintaining good health'*

7. What is the full meaning of GMC? What does GMC do?

'The GMC is the "General Medical Council". It is a body that has a statutory duty to maintain the registration of medical practitioners within the UK. The main roles that the GMC undertakes are:

- *Registering doctors to practise with provisional or full licences*

- *Setting standards for practice*

- *Dealing with concerns about whether a doctor is attaining the set standards for practice*

- *Running quality assurance of Medicine degrees within the UK to ensure the necessary standards are met'*

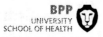

8. **Give an example of someone who has been struck off the GMC register.**

> *'A widely publicised case of a doctor being struck off the GMC register was that of Andrew Wakefield in 2010. The decision was reached by a tribunal of the GMC in relation to a now discredited claim advocated by Wakefield in 1998 that there is a link between receiving the MMR vaccine and acquiring bowel disease and autism. He was found by the tribunal to have acted "dishonestly and irresponsibly" in his published research, as well as acting against the interests of his patients and having "failed in his duties as a responsible consultant". His fraudulent research paper led to a big decrease in the uptake of the MMR vaccine and therefore put hundreds of thousands of people's health at risk. Andrew Wakefield is now banned from practising Medicine in the UK.'*

9. **How have the 'recent' reforms changed the NHS?**

This is an example of a question that was topical at the time of our interviews. The answer gives you an idea as to what level you should understand the key changes to the NHS. At the time of writing, topical questions will include the junior doctor contracts and strikes.

The 'Health and Social Care Act 2012' greatly changed the structure of the NHS, giving 'clinical commissioning groups' (led by GP consortia) the majority of the NHS budget to commission services to their patients. This policy eliminated Primary Care Trusts (PCTs) and Strategic Health Authorities (SHAs). There are several arguments for the pros and cons of these reforms.

Pros include:

- GPs are allowed to shape how services are provided. They can choose to allocate more resources into treatment for a specific disease that may be more prevalent in their area.

- If GPs aren't paid any more money, the NHS saves money as they do not have to pay the PCT/SHA managers.

Cons include:

- GP waiting lists may get longer as GPs are responsible for commissioning care as well as practising Medicine.

- GPs may lack the expertise in commissioning care, and so GP consortia may end up hiring the managers from the abolished PCTs.

> ***Overall***: *A wait and see approach must be taken in this case, as it is impossible to predict how effective these reforms will be. A lot of money may be saved through less management, but equally billions of pounds are being spent on restructuring the NHS and retraining staff.*
>
> *The recent NHS reforms have drastically changed the structure of the NHS, abolishing PCTs and SHAs whilst giving the majority of the budget to GP consortia. The main advantages are that GPs can shape the treatment they provide to match the needs of the patients in their area, and that abolishing PCTs should save management costs. However, GPs lack the expertise in commissioning care and may have to hire the managers who worked for PCTs, and thus money would not be saved. Overall, the effects of the reforms will not be fully known for a few years yet. Money may be saved from a reduction in management costs, but equally money spent on restructuring and retraining may be lost.*

10. **Due to budget cutbacks there are limited resources within the NHS; what would you do to save money?**

    There are a number of areas in which money could potentially be saved within the NHS. It is important when answering this question that you reflect upon not only the benefits, but also the flaws of cutting back resources in a particular area. Here are some ways money could be saved:

    - **Homeopathic medicine** – the use of homeopathic medicine within the NHS is quite controversial, as it does not conform to the usual evidence based practice required for other drugs within the NHS. Cutting the use of these medicines could save the NHS millions of pounds a year, but it would reduce 'patient choice' available.

    - **Missed appointments** – missed appointments cost the NHS hundreds of millions of pounds a year. Asking people to pay a small fee if they did not attend (DNA) could cut down the amount of missed appointments and provide a financial windfall from those that are still missed. However, this could place financial strain on patients who cannot afford those fees.

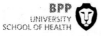

- **Limit non-essential services** – if some services are under-used in a local area, they could be merged together to save costs, or the hours could be cut.

- **Prevention rather than cure** – treatment of patients costs much more than preventative measures early on. Focusing on prevention can save a significant amount of money.

    - Include big and small savings that will add up over time

    - Explain the benefits but include pitfalls

    - Draw upon your wider reading to show your understanding

---

'Saving money is a vital issue for the NHS. One way to do this could be cutting back the use of homeopathy, as it isn't supported by evidence based medicine. However, this could limit patient choice. In addition, a small contribution could be introduced for missed appointments as this wastes hundreds of millions of pounds of the NHS budget each year. However, this could place a financial strain on lower income patients. Also, under-used local services could be merged to cut back on costs, though this could mean patients have to travel further for treatment. However, I believe the best way for the NHS to save more money in the long run is to focus on preventing diseases as this approach is a lot cheaper than treatment.'

---

11. What's your view on the European Working Time Directive?

Since 2009, the European Working Time Directive (EWTD) has restricted the number of hours people in Europe can work. The main measures of the EWTD are:

- The average working week must be 48 hours or less.

- There must be a daily rest of 11 hours per 24-hour period.

- There must be right to a day off each week.

- There must be right to a rest break if the working day is longer than six hours.

Doctors can 'opt out' of the directive and work longer hours. There are many pros and cons of the EWTD and it is important that you make a balanced argument.

Pros include:

- The EWTD ensures that doctors are fresh and alert when treating patients resulting in improved patient care and lowering the chances of a mistake being made.

- Some argue that working 48 hours a week gives junior doctors sufficient training and that working longer periods doesn't add to their expertise in treating patients.

Cons include:

- The EWTD means there is a lack of continuity of care for patients. Instead of seeing two or three doctors during a stay at hospital, they are seeing five or six. This leaves more room for errors in communication during handovers, so the most effective treatment may not always be carried out.

- Some argue that by reducing the amount of time junior doctors are working they will be less experienced and therefore in the future consultants will be less qualified. This may lead to standards of patient care by doctors dropping.

  – Explain the EWTD
  – Give the pros and cons
  – Conclude with a balanced view

'Due to the European Working Time Directive, doctors cannot work longer than 48 hours per week with at least 11 hours' rest per 24 hours and a full 24 hours' uninterrupted rest per week. However, doctors are allowed to opt out of the 48-hour limit and can be "on call" in case of emergencies for long periods of unsociable hours.

An advantage of this is that doctors should be more alert whilst working and provide a higher standard of care. However, it may result in a lack of continuity of care if doctors work shorter shifts more frequently. It is also argued that junior doctors require long working times in order to receive adequate training. Overall, I feel the EWTD is useful as doctors working excessively long hours are more prone to make mistakes, and those doctors that want to can opt out of the 48-hour limit.'

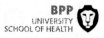

12. How did the NHS start?

As the NHS will be the employer of 99% of Medicine graduates it is good to show the interviewers that you have done some research into the NHS and its beginnings.

The 'National Insurance Act 1911' ensured that in exchange for contributions from their pay check workers were entitled to medical care, but not necessarily to the drugs needed. There was a consensus prior to World War II that reform was needed with dependants also receiving health insurance, and that different types of hospitals should be integrated. However, due to the start of WWII, no action was taken.

The post-war reconstruction gave an opportunity, which might not have been possible in peacetime, for an NHS to be set up. The 'Beveridge Report' of 1942 identified disease as being one of the 'Five Giant Evils' as it prevented men from working and therefore caused financial problems. The report gained bipartisan and massive public support. In 1945, following Labour's election victory, multiple social policies, known as the 'Welfare State', were introduced, including the 'National Health Service Act 1946', which laid the foundations for the NHS's formation.

The NHS was finally launched on 5th July 1948 with three core principles:

- To meet the needs of everybody
- To be free at the point of delivery
- To be based on clinical need, not ability to pay

'The NHS began in 1948 following the "National Health Service Act 1946". Disease had been named as one of the "Five Great Evils" that the Government should combat in the Beveridge Report in 1942, as it prevented people from working and therefore caused financial problems. This report gained widespread support from the public and major political parties. Therefore, during reconstruction after the Second World War setting up an NHS was a priority for the new Labour Government. The NHS was launched in 1948 with three core principles; to meet the needs of everybody; to be free at the point of delivery; and to be based on clinical need, not ability to pay.'

13. Outline what you know of postgraduate training.

- In general, degrees for undergraduates in Medicine last five or six years. However, once a student has graduated they must spend a significant amount of time in training before they become a General Practitioner (GP), a Consultant, or a Staff Grade doctor.

- Training to become a GP or Consultant takes differing amounts of time, but all Medicine graduates wishing to become a doctor must first complete two years of training as a 'Foundation Doctor'. In the first year (FY1), you will rotate through three or four jobs in different specialities. The year builds upon the training and skills learnt as an undergraduate. In the second year (FY2), you will do further posts in different specialities and build upon competencies learnt in the first year.

- The next stage to becoming a GP or Consultant, following your two years as a Foundation Doctor, is to become a 'Specialist Registrar'. Those wishing to become a GP will do three years in general practice, and those wishing to become a Consultant will generally do a minimum of six/ seven years in a hospital speciality. Specialist Registrars will take part in structured training programmes directly after their completion of their foundation years.

- Overall, this means that following your undergraduate training you must do a minimum of a further eight years' training to become a Consultant and five years to become a GP.

'After completion of Medical School, you firstly must complete two years of training as a foundation doctor. During these years you will rotate among various specialties and build upon competencies acquired at Medical School. After your foundation programme you will become a specialist registrar, at which time you will have to decide which path you will take: either staying in a hospital environment or moving to general practice. Becoming a consultant requires a minimum of six further years of training and to become a GP requires three further years, so in total this is a minimum of eight years and five years respectively after graduating from Medical School.'

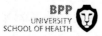
BPP
UNIVERSITY
SCHOOL OF HEALTH

Work experience / Wider reading

1. What are the roles of a doctor?

2. How do you know Medicine is the right career for you?

3. What have you read or experienced in order to prepare you for Medicine?

4. What did you learn about yourself from your work experience?

5. How do you keep up with medical issues?

6. What have you seen in the news recently that has interested you?

7. Who was in the MDT meeting that you observed?

8. Who is the most important member of a medical team?

9. How do the media portray doctors?

1. **What are the roles of a doctor?**

There are many different roles that a doctor is required to undertake. Here are some examples of the changing role of a doctor:

- **Listener:** Doctors have to listen well to take an accurate history.

- **Team player:** Doctors work as team players when treating patients. Whether it's part of a surgical team or in a multidisciplinary team (MDT), there are lots of situations where doctors must work well in a team.

- **Leader/manager:** Doctors lead the decision-making on what action to take with a patient, and lead the team that treats them.

- **Educator:** Junior doctors teach their contemporaries and medical students, and senior doctors undertake teaching at Medical Schools and university hospitals.

  - Listener
  - Role in teams (team member and team leader)
  - Educator

> *'There are many different roles that a doctor must undertake. A doctor must be a good listener when diagnosing a patient, ensuring they don't miss any symptoms of a serious illness. Being a team player is another role a doctor must undertake. In MDT meetings a doctor must work well with their colleagues to ensure the best treatment is pursued for the patient. Finally, being an educator is another role of doctors, passing on their knowledge and skills to fellow and future doctors.'*

2. **How do you know Medicine is the right career for you?**

Interviewers will want to know that you have taken careful consideration in your choice to become a doctor, and that it isn't something that you have decided on a whim. This can be demonstrated by activities that you have undertaken such as:

- Work experience
- Talking to medical students and doctors
- Reading medical journals/books

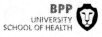

> *'Having initially been inspired to study Medicine following my successful maxillofacial surgery, I undertook work shadowing to give me a further insight into what being a doctor entails. This allowed me to discuss with various doctors about pursuing a career in Medicine. Furthermore, the care and compassion shown to patients during my shadowing was absolutely compelling and reaffirmed my commitment to Medicine.'*

3. **What have you read or experienced in order to prepare you for Medicine?**

   This is designed to make sure you've really researched the profession. Do not say you've read something when you haven't!

   - Be honest
   - Re-read things close to the interviews
   - Be able to talk about the books intelligibly

> *'I have read a few books about Medicine and the jobs a doctor has to perform specifically as a Junior Doctor. The books that had the biggest effect on me were; "The Rise and Fall of Modern Medicine" by Le Fanu and "Trust Me I'm a Junior Doctor" by Max Pemberton. Le Fanu's was a fascinating book about Medicine's recent progression. However, I didn't really agree with the author's belief that Medicine couldn't advance any more, especially with so many diseases still having no cure and the constant development in medical techniques being made. Pemberton's was a humorous book that showed me some of the trials and tribulations I would face on my path to become a doctor. The book showed that becoming a doctor is tough and there are many unglamorous and daunting tasks I would have to perform. Wanting to learn and understand more about Medicine, I enthusiastically undertook work experience in both a Paediatric and an Oncology Ward. They were both fantastic experiences for me as I saw how a hospital runs and the variety of jobs doctors must do. I also spent my time there talking to doctors, young and old, about their experiences.'*

4. **What did you learn about yourself from your work experience?**

   It is important to demonstrate that you have learnt a lot from your work experience, and made the maximum possible use of your opportunity to undertake work experience. Use self-awareness and assess what you do well at the moment (such as communication with adults and older people) and what you need to do better (such as communication with children). Another thing to mention may be how coming into contact with seriously ill patients has affected you on a personal level. Most importantly, though, undertaking work experience should have the effect of confirming that Medicine is definitely the career path you are suited for. Include:

   • Work experience confirmed that Medicine is what you want to do

   • Things that stood out during your work experience

   • Your strengths and weaknesses, including room for improvement

   > 'Undertaking work experience at ... Hospital was not only a fascinating experience in understanding first-hand what being a doctor entails, but also allowed me to learn a lot about myself whilst I was there. Observing patients with incurable diseases such as Alzheimer's or cancer had a profound impact upon me, and demonstrated how essential it is to comfort patients. I also learnt to develop skills over the course of my shadowing, such as my communication with patients. Overall, the experiences I had reaffirmed that a career in Medicine is perfect for me and that I personally have the skills and qualities to one day become a good doctor.'

5. **How do you keep up with medical issues?**

   As a prospective medical student you are expected to have an interest in and keep up to date with current medical issues. There are numerous different sources available to keep up to date with the latest developments, including reading a magazine such as the *New Scientist* or *Student BMJ*, or a website such as BBC Health. If you mention reading a source regularly in your Personal Statement or interview, be prepared to answer questions about your reading.

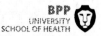

> 'I read Student BMJ every month in the local library, which gives good coverage of the most important medical news items. I watch the news most days, and if there is something medical I always follow up the story on BBC Health. I also like to read New Scientist, which keeps me informed.'

6. **What have you seen in the news recently that has interested you?**

Prior to attending an interview it is important to keep updated on the latest medical developments and to have a fairly good understanding of any big political/NHS issues that have been in the news. You could be asked about a specific recent medical issue or a topic of your choosing. Make sure you have a few topics you feel comfortable talking about.

A good format in which to answer this question is:

- Firstly, what is the issue you are talking about? How does it affect patients, staff and the NHS?

- Secondly, what is the recent development that has happened?

- Finally, what impact could this development have on treatment in the future?

7. **Who was in the MDT meeting that you observed?**

MDT meetings are an opportunity for experts in different specialities within healthcare to pool together their knowledge and experience in order to give patients the best possible treatment. Some people that you may expect to find at an MDT meeting include:

- Consultant surgeons
- Oncologists or other specialist doctors
- Radiographers
- Histologists
- Senior and specialist nurses
- Physiotherapists
- Social workers
- Any other relevant medical professionals

8. Who is the most important member of the medical team?

It is important not to overlook the contributions of other healthcare professionals; every team member is needed for good patient care.

- Mention doctors
- Mention nurses and other healthcare staff
- Refer to work experience to provide an example

'When treating a patient it is important to remember that medical staff work together as a team in order to treat the patient as effectively as possible. Doctors may have the ultimate responsibility for what treatment to pursue, but without nurses and carers administering the care the patient would have no hope of recovering. When performing an operation, the entire surgical team (surgeons, anaesthetists, nurses, etc) must work in harmony to ensure that the surgery is a success. Therefore, I would argue that there is no single most important member as the entire team depends on each and every team member fulfilling their role.'

9. How does the media portray doctors?

- Highlight good portrayal
- Highlight bad portrayal
- Give examples

'Some newspapers in the UK are sensationalist, giving very mixed views on doctors. In some stories, a newspaper may criticise doctors for being overpaid, and have negative stories about treatment of patients by doctors and doctors being struck off, for example Andrew Wakefield in 2010. In other stories, though, doctors are praised for developing new treatments and for their successful treatment of patients. In some TV shows such as "Grey's Anatomy", doctors are portrayed as being hard working and dedicated to their jobs; although the show can be described as overly dramatic, it also focuses a lot on the characters' personal lives (rather than them practising Medicine). In others, such as "Scrubs", doctors are portrayed as being less professional. Overall, the media portrays doctors in a very mixed light.'

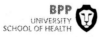

Ethics and law

1. What's your opinion on (ethical issue)?

2. In what circumstances would you perform abortions as a doctor?

3. A young girl comes into your GP surgery and asks to go on the pill. What would you do?

4. Would you give a smoker a lung transplant?

5. Is it justified to refuse a hip operation to an obese patient who has no medical reason for their obesity?

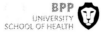

1. What's your opinion on (ethical issue)?

- Recognise it is an ethical issue
- Discuss the pros and cons of the issue
- Weigh everything up and come to a conclusion

Eg for euthanasia:

> *'This is an ethical dilemma. Euthanasia is currently illegal in this country. However, supporters of euthanasia argue that if a patient is able to choose how they are treated, the choice to die should be allowed too. Furthermore, they argue that it is not fair for doctors to allow patients to suffer when they could be allowed to have a dignified death. On the other side, opponents of euthanasia use the sanctity of life argument. Life is sacred; no man should have the power to take someone else's life. They also worry that legalising euthanasia will set a bad precedent and many people will see it as an 'easy way out', especially if encouraged by family members or friends. I personally feel euthanasia is wrong, although supporters do make some good points. My biggest concern would be if euthanasia were to be legalised it would be very difficult to regulate, and it could be the beginning of a "slippery slope".'*

2. In what circumstances would you perform abortions as a doctor?

Abortion is legal up to 24 weeks if two doctors are of the opinion that the mental or physical health of the mother or existing children of her family would be affected by the pregnancy. Abortion thereafter can only be carried out if:

- The abortion is required to prevent grave permanent injury to the physical/mental health of the mother

- By continuing the pregnancy the mother's life is at greater risk than having the abortion

- There's a high risk of the child having physical or mental abnormalities

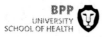

3. **A young girl comes into your GP surgery and asks to go on the pill. What would you do?**

   - Recognise it is an ethical issue

   - Go through the steps you would take before making a decision

   - Finally say what decision you would make

   > *'Firstly I would make sure the girl is competent and understands what she is asking for. I would then ask her reasons for wanting the pill, and ensure other people haven't coerced her into making the decision. Finally, I would advise her to confide in someone she trusts and see what he or she thinks and then come back to me. If she still wants to go through with it and I'm satisfied with her reasons and capacity I will give her the pill as well as explaining how the pill works and the possible side effects, and how to practise safe sex.'*

4. **Would you give a smoker a lung transplant?**

   A good way to think about questions based on transplants is to consider biology, psychology and society ...

   - **Biology**: How good a match are the donor and recipient, how old is the recipient (have to survive the operation and go through recovery), is recurrence of the problem inevitable?

   - **Psychology**: If self-inflicted (drinking/smoking) will this happen again, will the patient be compliant with immunosuppressant treatment?

   - **Society**: Does the donor have dependants, how does the donor contribute to society?

   It's important to consider all of the above, without prejudice or assumptions, in a multidisciplinary team meeting.

   - Recognise it is an ethical issue

   - Give reasons for and against

   - Conclude with how you would handle the issue and explain why

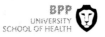

'This is an ethical dilemma. Doctors shouldn't judge a person on their background or lifestyle when treating them. Therefore some argue doctors shouldn't focus on the patient's smoking and should simply find a way to treat them, in this case giving them a new lung. However, others argue that it is unfair for non-smokers to be on level-pegging with smokers whose illness is self-inflicted. They say smokers should be put at the bottom of the transplant list and non-smokers should get the transplant first. I can see the reasoning behind both views. If I were faced with the situation I would help the patient to quit smoking, and if they actively try to stop I would go through with the transplant. However, if they don't try at all or fall into bad habits again I would give the lung to a non-smoker as the lungs will be likely to last longer.'

5. **Is it justified to refuse a hip operation for an obese patient who has no medical reason for their obesity?**

   - Recognise it is an ethical issue
   - Pros and cons for giving hip transplants to obese people
   - Conclude with what you think is the best thing to do

'This is an ethical problem. On the one hand, it could be seen as unfair to restrict treatment to obese people when doctors are still treating other self-inflicted illnesses. The main argument, however, is that a doctor should always do their best to help patients. Flat out refusing to help them just because they have a weight problem is out of the question. On the other hand, one could say it is wrong for people needing new hips such as the elderly to be behind people who have let themselves become obese. Giving new hips to the obese could set a bad precedent as others could think there's always treatment available so there's no need to change their bad habits. The best thing to do, in my opinion, is to allow obese people hip transplants, but only if they attempt to lose weight. So hopefully, after the transplant, they continue to work at losing weight.'

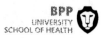

Academic

The following questions are just an example of what you could be asked:

- You studied 'Molecules, Medicines and Drugs' with the Open University. What do you understand of the difference between medicines and drugs?

- How is rejection prevented in transplants?

- Which of your school subjects interested you the most?

- Talk to me about a part of human biology that really interests you.

- What is HIV?

- What are the current most prevalent causes of death in the UK?

- Why does the body make you faint as a defence mechanism to lack of oxygen to the brain?

- How does an increase in heart rate cause an increase in blood pressure?

- What might cause a build-up of tissue fluid?

This list is infinite, but most interviews will not focus on these questions, because your academic knowledge is already presumed from your predicted and/or achieved grades. Your passion for science and Medicine should be the driving force you need to research and understand these topics. Even if questions are out of the scope of your school subject curricula, the wider reading that should be part of your weekly routine (BBC Health, newspapers, journals/magazines etc) should give you a good enough grounding to answer these with confidence.

It's important that you feel confident talking about any medical condition you have mentioned in your Personal Statement. Also be able to explain any recent medical developments, and try to bring in anything you have learned during your Biology/Chemistry/Physics courses if relevant to the question asked.

- What relevance to Medicine are the A Levels / (Advanced) Highers, apart from Biology and Chemistry, which you have been studying?

BPP
UNIVERSITY
SCHOOL OF HEALTH

Your answer to this question will obviously depend on what subjects you are studying. Here are some skills that different subjects bring to the table:

- Foreign Languages (communication, self-study skills, group work)

- Music/Art/Drama (stress release, observation/listening skills)

- Maths/Physics (logical thought, mental agility)

- Physical Education (teamwork, motivation, competition)

- English and Humanities (writing, analytical skills)

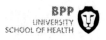

Oxbridge

For many students, Oxford or Cambridge is the dream. If you are one of these students, you will have to work harder than ever before to ensure your dream is achieved.

Oxbridge interviews are unique and intense – you will be pushed to your limit. Questions can delve into any theme the interviewers fancy. You can have numerous interviews, in various colleges.

In the past, students were given a medical article to read shortly before their interview, on which they are tested.

Questions based on the article may include:

- What is this article about?
- Do you think the article is biased? Who is it in favour of?
- Sum each paragraph up in one sentence.

You will be asked scientific questions based on your Personal Statement. For example, if you've mentioned a book you've read, or a favourite journal, be prepared to talk at length about the content, including recent and older articles if you've mentioned a medical/scientific journal.

Throughout the interviews at Oxbridge you will have to display: a logical thought process, clarity of expression, and an ability to defend your arguments.

You will likely be wrong at times, but this is OK. Oxbridge interviews are not about simple regurgitation, but rather lateral thinking. This will be novel for you, and the interviewer will be there to push you along.

There are whole books on the Oxbridge application and interview process. Refer to these, ask friends who've applied in the past, and talk to current students. Courses are also available.

We would recommend that you note down the points you made during your BMAT essay. This will likely form part of the interview.

Oxbridge tutors will be keen to see that you will be an asset to their college. Ensure you mention what you can bring to their college and how you will contribute to its community as well.

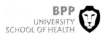

Here are some example questions that should give you an idea of what you could be asked:

- How would you design a brain?

- What causes Down's syndrome?

- Is the baby of a mother with HIV more likely to get HIV during natural childbirth or through a caesarean section?

- How would you go about creating a vaccine for HIV?

- Suppose a vaccine has made it through animal trials, how would you go about testing whether it's safe and effective for humans?

- Does our brain give us an accurate representation of the world?

- What is the skin made up of? What about scar tissue?

- What is the Polypill? Should we use it?

- What is the molecular mass of haemoglobin and how many iron atoms does it have?

- How do ears work?

- How do blood pressure monitors work?

- If you were going to categorise diseases where would you start?

- What do you know about the pituitary gland?

- What is autism and how might oxytocin be related to it?

- How is the volume of blood in the body calculated?

- Why do we inherit diseases and shouldn't evolution prevent this?

- The cause of cystic fibrosis is related to a mutation in a gene that codes for which protein?

- Here is a picture of a... What is wrong with it?

- Why are cancer cells more susceptible to radiation than normal cells?

You cannot prepare for every single question – the interviewers have free reign, and each and every interview will be individual.

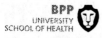

What you can do is tackle problems logically and sensitively – being clear, concise and coherent.

Try to enjoy your interview, and don't be upset if you feel the panel is pushing you or you don't know an answer. They may act as the Devil's advocate. That's their job!

If you don't know the answer to something, ask! Show interest into finding out the answer.

Be enthusiastic, logical and smile!

Good luck!

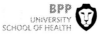

Problem-Based Learning (PBL)

PBL is used in most Medical Schools, so it is important that you can describe what it is ...

PBL was pioneered at McMaster University, Canada, in 1969. PBL has been described as: 'Any learning environment in which the problem drives the learning.' (Dr Woods, McMaster University). PBL involves small group work and self-directed learning.

There is a chair who leads the session, a scribe who notes down information and questions, and a facilitator who guides the session if needs be. Students start by reading through a 'case' together. They explore existing knowledge and scribe this down, alongside key information from the case. The group then formulates questions for self-study: what do you need to know, what should you go over, what's the best thing to do for the patient etc. The group then spends a few hours researching the topic on their own before meeting up again to discuss their findings. Students should draw upon a wide range of materials and discussion should be fruitful and interactive. Everyone should participate. The end result is a reinforcement of learning and a conclusion for the case: what should be done for this patient.

Medical Schools can ask:

1. **What do you know about PBL?**

'*PBL was developed at McMaster Medical School in Canada about 50 years ago. The tutor of the PBL group provides a clinical case study, which becomes the focus of study for the group. The first task will be to brainstorm the topics with knowledge already possessed. Each student will then either work on one part of the problem, which is decided at the initial meeting, or every student will tackle every issue. After a period of self-study, the group meets and each member shares their findings. They will try to find the best way forward for that case. During both sessions a chair leads the group, giving direction and managing time, and a scribe works in the background recording the discussion.*'

2. What are the advantages/disadvantages of PBL?

'The advantages of PBL are: it develops your team-working, communication and independent learning skills, all essential for a doctor; you get to share your thoughts with the rest of the group, and get to hear what others have to say, which reinforces your learning (and you might understand their explanation better); you learn in a group, which reflects life as a doctor in a multidisciplinary team.

The disadvantages of PBL are: if you don't get along with some of the group members it could disrupt your learning; it may not be the best learning technique for you; you may not go into the same depth as you would in more traditional/integrated courses.'

3. Have you had any experience of independent learning?

'I have had experience of independent learning. I undertook an Open University course over the summer whilst in 6th form, entitled "Molecules, Medicines and Drugs: A Chemical Story". I believe it was my self-starter attitude that allowed me to excel at the course. It taught me a lot, not only about the science behind everyday drugs, but also about the dedication required for Higher Education study.'

4. What previous experience have you had learning in a small group?

'I took Spanish as one of my A Level choices. There were only five of us in my class. We often did group work and my teamwork skills improved immeasurably. We shared thoughts, bounced ideas off one another, and all worked to try to improve our understanding of the language.'

5. Why do you think PBL will suit you?

'I think PBL will suit me because I'm very motivated and I enjoy working in a group. I think PBL will actually take me out of my comfort zone, because most of the learning during high school is "spoon-fed", and in turn this "new" style of learning will make me into a better doctor. I'm under no illusion of the responsibility placed on each team member, and look forward to being able to contribute and learn from others.'

Multiple Mini Interviews (MMI)

Multiple Mini Interviews (MMI) were piloted in the UK at St George's Medical School, London, as a replacement for the traditional interview. It was felt that it was a fairer process, because if one station goes badly, you have other chances to redeem yourself. Also, it allows the interviewers to really test your communication skills, as you have to participate in role-plays, which cannot be rehearsed for. Another reason for introducing MMI was that it allows more candidates to be tested simultaneously, ensuring a faster process and reducing the number of interviewers required. Instead of taking a candidate's word for it, the admissions team can put skills to the test.

The most important reason to use MMI is to give universities the chance to test your communication skills, which cannot be assessed in the Personal Statement or in your Reference.

Several stations are used, lasting five to ten minutes each. A buzzer sounds, and you then have to move to the next station. It is important that you take a breather between stations, and do your best to forget what you just went through and focus on the station you are at.

An example MMI session could be:

1. **Organ donation**

   Views on 'opt in' and opt out'. Then a few scenarios: who should get a transplant?

2. **Alcoholic friend role-play**

   'Your friend has recently spent a night in A&E after a night out. Her parents are worried and want you to speak to her. You have to find out the severity of her drinking problem and work out a way forward together.'

3. **Internet self-diagnosis role-play**

   'Your friend has self-diagnosed himself on the internet, and thinks he has a serious condition. His symptoms are … . He wants your advice.'

MMIs and their role in the application process are explained below by Dr Dipak Kanabar, Sub Dean of Admissions (Medicine) at King's College London.

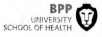

'At King's we used to employ a traditional 2:1 format of interview. We invited applicants into an interview room for a 20-minute period of assessment of their skills and aptitude to Medicine. Two assessors (clinical and preclinical) would ask questions in a standard format and score the candidate. We then ranked the candidate in order of their performance, before making an offer.

MMI interviews are increasingly being recognised as a fairer way of assessing a prospective candidate applying to Medicine. They have recently been introduced at King's and have proved successful in a number of ways. Post-MMI debriefs indicate that applicants feel less nervous and find the process of interview a lot more structured. Each candidate will pass through a series of stations lasting 5–10 minutes and be presented with a different scenario with a short break in between stations. Candidates report that the 90-second break in between each MMI station gives them an opportunity to recover their thoughts and prepare with a "fresh mind set" for the next station.

MMIs should be approached with the view that although a candidate should attempt to do well in all stations, in fact very few candidates manage this. Each station has a different assessor and marking scheme, and the candidate should use the 90-second break to try and forget about what they should have just said (or what they forgot to say) in the previous station, and try and focus on the next station and anticipate the range of questions or analysis of data/information about to be presented to them.

Candidates should attempt to set up MMI panels in their schools / A Level colleges and get used to the idea of timed questions with short breaks and a range of different interviewers. Most A Level students should be able to organise this amongst themselves and, as MMIs are increasingly being used in a variety of interview applications (nursing, pharmacy, dentistry etc), it is possible for groups of students at the same school to get together to organise mock MMI interviews in their school hall covering a range of disciplines. Remember that the caring professions are often all looking for the same qualities of professionalism; time management; empathy; good values and critical thinking.

A good candidate should pay attention to the task and/or listen carefully to the question. Before answering, they should quickly assimilate any available information in their minds, and then formulate a structure of answering the question in a logical way, before saying a word –

remember the considered response can often impress. We assess a variety of skills at MMI including considering ethical dilemmas; assessing communication skills and critical thinking; solving a problem; assessing values, skills and aptitudes; and data analysis.

My best advice: Remember that we have invited you (the candidate) to interview on the basis of your achievements and performance thus far. Be confident that you are amongst the select few being invited from the thousands of applications we receive each year. At King's one of our mottoes is "Distinguish yourself" and the MMI is your opportunity to tell us more about yourself and why you believe we should select you from hundreds of others competing with you for a place to read Medicine. Try and prepare by setting up an MMI mock interview in your school hall with your school friends and other prospective applicants – this will highlight the importance of timing your thinking and talking to a 5-minute period of MMI station assessment. Finally, listen carefully to what is being asked of you. Our MMI stations are not designed to trick or fool you; we wish to bring out the best in you so that you can demonstrate to us that you will not only be a successful undergraduate, but will also flourish as an outstanding practicing clinician in the future.'

4. Dead pet role-play

'Your neighbour left her guinea pig with you when she went on holiday. You looked after it well, but through no fault of your own the pet passed away. The lady opposite is your neighbour. You have to tell her what's happened.'

How to break bad news

- Set the scene (sit down in a quiet place, use a soft tone)
- Say explicitly that you have bad news
- Explain what has happened, give them time to take this in
- Don't interrupt when they respond
- Apologise, and see if there is anything that you can do

5. The NHS

Tell me about the NHS. What does it do well? What could be better? Would you consider working in the private sector?

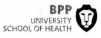

6. **Punishments for Medical Students**

   How should a student who ... be punished?

   - Plagiarises an essay
   - Tells a friend the contents of an exam
   - Steals a library book
   - Cheats during an exam

   A list of punishments is given, and you then have to explain which punishment you would give and why.

7. **Making a storyline with a partner**

   You have a number of pictures, which form a story, and your partner has the rest. You have to work together to create the story, without looking at each other's set (placing them face down in order). The only way to work out the order is by spotting small clues in each image, which then leads to the next.

   You may be asked how this went, and what you could have done better.

8. **Sad stranger**

   'You arrive at your regular bus stop and find a stranger crying. What will you do?'

9. **Observing a consultation**

   You might be asked to observe a doctor talking to a patient.

   You would then be asked to comment on how you think the consultation went. Include things that could be improved, eg the doctor being more empathetic, the patient being more involved in decision-making, and highlight what went well, eg the doctor showing active listening.

MMI was designed to test the following: empathy, problem-solving skills, ethical reasoning and your communication skills. Ensure you put these skills across.

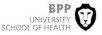

Problem solving

Some schools present students with mental problems and give some time for students to work out a solution. Don't get too worked up about getting the correct answer. In these situations the interviewer is more interested in a logical thought process.

There isn't really much revision you can do for something like this but trying to think clearly and show clear working often earns you brownie points.

Group interviews

Some Medical Schools use a similar process to MMI, but start with a group interview. The discussion is based on an ethical dilemma and you have to talk it through together. It's important to show good teamwork and communication skills. If people aren't saying much, try to include them in the discussion and ensure you don't dominate proceedings (but you can lead!).

Practice makes perfect

We would urge you to try to establish a mock MMI event with fellow applicants in your college or local area. You can all plan stations assessing different skillsets, and then take it in turns to undertake the stations. This way you can act as both interviewee and judge. This 'mock' session will let you practise the timings, and encourage you to develop quick and flexible thinking.

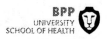

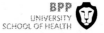

Chapter 5
Surviving Medical School

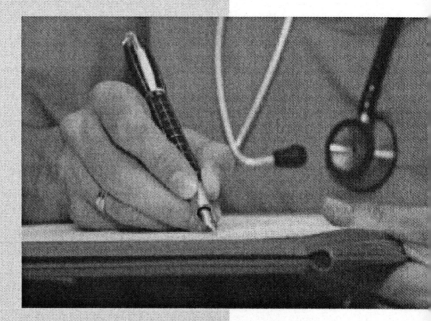

Starting at Medical School

You've made it!

Congratulations for getting a place in one of the most competitive subjects at university. They said the hard part was getting in! However, your work doesn't stop here; it is imperative to maintain the momentum you have built up through the application process. A number of students perform badly and some have to leave Medical School due to losing track of their goal. Of course that doesn't mean you work day and night throughout term, but it does mean that you follow a routine and have a sensible 'work-life balance'.

So what should you be doing once at Medical School?

The aim of this chapter is not to tell you what you can and can't do but rather to give some tips and guidance. While applying to Medical School many of us have programmed ourselves to be leaders in everything that crosses our path. We embrace every opportunity with open arms and can't get enough of juggling activities with our workload. It's great to be an all-rounder and partaking in things other than work will keep you well balanced. Nevertheless, many students will tell you that university, and particularly Medical School, is a different ball game and one must adapt.

A common experience for many first years is to get involved with every activity being flaunted. By all means have a taster of what's on offer but remember that the time you can devote is limited.

Key Point:

Try new things and continue with old hobbies, but remember why you're there!

Accommodation

Research accommodation early. As soon as you get an offer have a serious think and apply early. Try to attend Open Days initially and Post-Offer Visit Days if you can, and have a look around the accommodation on offer. Most first year students are guaranteed university accommodation.

The main choice is whether you want to live in self-catered or catered accommodation ('halls'). Some people enjoy cooking for themselves in self-catered accommodation, which works out a lot cheaper. Others prefer halls where food is provided, and it offers you a great chance to meet lots of new people.

> **Key Point:**
>
> Do your homework and apply early.

Important considerations are price, facilities and location. Research these via Accommodation Services.

Freshers'/Introduction/Welcome Week

Enjoy yourself and try to experience everything you can. Meet as many people as you can and enjoy yourself!

Take advantage of the deals and offers for students; many will last during the year. Don't settle for the first event waved in your face, there will be something you like, so look around. Join the social networking groups for your university. Many students post their accommodation offers online and this gives them a head start in networking with fellow first years.

> **Key Point:**
>
> Make the most of your Freshers' Week. You're only a Fresher once!

Starting the course

The workload is not very demanding at the start of term. This is deliberate as a way of easing students into the course.

Although it might seem over-the-top, try to create a timetable and begin to work to a routine to avoid the pressure building up and finding yourself sinking in a vicious cycle.

> **Key Point:**
>
> Get into good habits early.

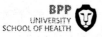

Sports

From past experience as a fresher keen to meet new people and network within the Medical School, sports teams are brilliant starting points. There are the traditional medical sports such as rugby, hockey, football and cricket. If you cannot find the medical sports team of your choice there are usually a variety of general university sports teams to fill that void, or set up a new medical sports team yourself!

Most Medical Schools have their own sports teams and joining these can secure a network of older students who you can bug with queries and often receive useful resources from pre-exams! Of course, if you don't enjoy sports there are several other opportunities; however, don't be intimidated about skill level, as there are usually teams of mixed ability.

There are also the social teams, which as you've guessed are more about after-match socials rather than the games themselves but nonetheless cater for every medic and are usually the starting point if you are a newbie to the sport. This is the option for relaxed individuals looking for more of a 'fun' time.

Being part of a sports team or activity not only allows you to meet new people but it also contributes to your health and wellbeing. Student life can be stressful; this coupled with an unhealthy student diet may result in your health and wellbeing suffering. Hence regular exercise and playing sport can provide a long-term opportunity to keep fit and stay healthy.

> ### *Key Point:*
> Get involved with a sports team whatever your level. Do not be afraid to try a new sport.

Societies and activities

Get involved with societies and activities you enjoy. You can't just be studying 24 hours a day! Societies are great not just for gaining valuable experiences but also for meeting new people. Getting to know students in years above is a big help. You will find numerous fun activities to choose from such as:

• Drama/Musical groups

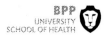

- Dance societies
- Faith/Cultural societies
- Humanitarian groups
- Debating groups

If you have an interest that's not accommodated for by a society, set a new one up!

> ## Key Point:
>
> Have a look at the activities on offer and join ones that you find enjoyable.

Medical Society (MedSoc)

Joining the Medical Society (MedSoc) at university is a good idea. Most first year medics do join their MedSoc and go to their Fresher events. MedSoc provides another welcome networking opportunity during Freshers' and beyond.

> ## Key Point:
>
> Be part of your university Medical Society.

What textbooks do I need for the first year?

Each Medical School will have their recommended texts for different parts of the course.

It's a good idea to ask older years about books. They will know what you really need, or if it's just easier to occasionally borrow them from the library.

Universities may offer e-books online, so check with the library to see if this resource is available.

Instead of purchasing a new book, you could see if any friends/ family have finished with their medical books if you know anyone, or you can get some great deals in charity shops early in term. Older students also advertise books they want to sell on so keep your eye out for bargains.

If you do want to buy a new textbook, try it out in the library first to ensure you like it, comparing to other similar books.

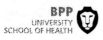
BPP
UNIVERSITY
SCHOOL OF HEALTH

Staying in Medical School

Accommodation

Living with medics after the first year has its perks; you have buddies to practise your newly acquired practical skills for OSCE exams with, for example, and they are often your closest friends.

However, staying with non-medics will help to keep you grounded and gives you a break from Medicine!

The downside of living with non-medics is that their timetables are not usually as taxing as yours and you may be disrupted by their social activities, particularly if they don't understand the demands of your work.

> ### *Key Point:*
> Think carefully about where and whom you would like to live with during your time at Medical School.

Support at Medical School

It is a good idea to establish a support network while at university. Most students are assigned a Personal Tutor / Director of Studies and you should realise that they really are there to help you! Talk to them about any issues that may require support, such as finance. There will be other support/advice services at your university too. Don't forget to register with a local GP.

> ### *Key Point:*
> Liaise with your Personal Tutor / Director of Studies and register with a local GP.

How much extra work should I be doing every day?

This is a common question and to be honest there is no set answer. Most universities and tutors give a benchmark for students. This can be anything from two to four hours a day depending on the period. It is advisable to spend time going over teaching which you have received for the day and to look at any forthcoming

BPP
UNIVERSITY
SCHOOL OF HEALTH

teaching topics. This will ensure you do not fall behind and at the same time reinforce the contents of topics.

Many students tend to ignore some categories of teaching, thinking of them as diluted material and not 'real' lectures, but the truth is they carry importance along with the usual physiology and anatomy subjects and will be examined.

> **Key Point:**
>
> Get into a good learning routine.

How should I revise for anatomy?

We have all been there and getting to grips with anatomy is akin to learning a new language! As with anything, anatomy requires time and practice. There are a number of methods that can be employed to aid revision.

- Pay attention during anatomy teaching.

- Use anatomy colouring books.

- Buy or rent a model skeleton.

- Dissection and prosection are very practical ways of learning and all too often students regret not having concentrated during these teaching sessions. As the resource is rather scarce, teaching tends to be delivered in groups so be sure to fully engage and ask questions.

- Ask your lecturer for help if you're really stuck.

> **Key Point:**
>
> Stick with it – it becomes easier the more time you spend on it! Ask for help if needed.

What should I do if activities are getting too much for me?

Say no! Yes, it really is that simple. When it comes to a point where you aren't able to revise because as Publicity Officer of the CoffeeSoc you have to email all the members about your latest coffee meeting you should think carefully about how much involvement is appropriate!

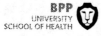
BPP
UNIVERSITY
SCHOOL OF HEALTH

As students and particularly future doctors, many of us feel ashamed to surrender or admit defeat in something we are involved in. Sometimes you need to take time out to think about what really matters. Positions in societies are great for personal and professional development, but you need to prioritise.

If there is an activity that is taking too much out of you, tell your peers that you really do have to concentrate on your studies.

Key Point:

Prioritise – do not let activities rule your life.

How do I complete a medical research project?

For many students taking part in a student selected module, this will be their first opportunity to write a medical essay or report. The first project will often involve getting used to reading medical journals, medical terminology and medical databases online.

A key resource is MedLine/PubMed, an online medical database of research papers, which will be your port of call for analysing previous research in your area of interest. Google Scholar is also an invaluable tool for searching for research papers.

There are often support sessions run by schools where students are taught about new techniques to conducting research. It takes time to get used to some of these new tools and as a result some students often resort to online search engines such as Google. Although these are good for a broad overview of the subject, learning how to use the more advanced tools in mainstream medical databases will stand you in good stead for the future and help when collecting references.

Remember to save your results, as you can go back to these to run searches again. A lot of time and effort is wasted when not writing references at the time of reading. Having well-referenced work is an important part of your research work and contributes to your assessment marks.

Always follow your university guidelines as to how they want the report to be presented, bearing in mind details such as word count, number of figures, size of font and line spacing.

BPP
UNIVERSITY
SCHOOL OF HEALTH

Never plagiarise! You may have gotten away with this in school (hopefully not!) but as you are now young doctors in the making you are expected to act as such. Medical Schools employ services such as Turnitin, which compares your work with all other students' work worldwide. Tutors can easily determine what is your work and what isn't. It is better to produce something of your own rather than getting a zero for a piece of work which has been copied from a website. Plagiarising may also put your place at Medical School in jeopardy and could tarnish your student record, which will be damaging to job prospects.

> ### *Key Point:*
>
> Don't leave it to the last minute. Finish and hand work in on time. Follow the recommended guidelines and do your own work.

I got a really low mark in my assessment, what do I do?

Ask for feedback. It is often the case that as students we shy away from this and as a result are left at the end of the year with unanswered questions, which can be quite easily solved by asking a brief question. It is also important to be honest and ask yourself if you have put enough effort in.

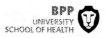

Building your Medical CV

It's important to start to build your Medical Portfolio throughout your time at Medical School, in addition to the standard teaching and learning expected and your social life.

Academically, you can attend lectures put on by the university, enter competitions, attend conferences or courses, produce and present a poster, publish some research, take part in summer research projects, and write articles for medical journals.

Although this may seem daunting, it is easier doing the above in your early years, before the workload and demands become greater still. Wait until you've settled in and then see if you can try something new and learn a transferable skill.

Being a part of a society shows commitment and if you get involved with the running of the society you can display team working, leadership and communication skills, as well as learning new skills and having fun!

Other things you can include are: travel, peer mentoring schemes, any voluntary work you do, any prizes you receive, any teaching experience you have and any capacity where you act as a leader, eg sport captaincy. Don't forget about part-time work, as this shows an ability to manage your time well and you learn transferable skills.

Try to keep a record of anything you do that's above and beyond the curriculum.

You may be asked by your Personal Tutor / Director of Studies to send them your CV. This gives you a good chance to keep it current and ensure you don't forget anything! Even if they don't request one, you could ask if they wouldn't mind checking through it, and they can give you some good hints and tips and general advice so you can appropriately record your achievements, which will really help in later years.

Medical Organisations

What organisations should I join as a medical student?

There are a number of organisations you will meet during Freshers' and beyond. It is important to join a medical indemnity provider such as the Medical Defence Union or Medical Protection Service. These organisations protect you should something go wrong during Medical School placements and electives. As a doctor you will continue to use these services but pay for them, so take advantage of the student rates while you can.

Medical Defence Union website: www.themdu.com

Medical Protection Service website: www.medicalprotection.org/uk

MDDUS (Scotland) website: www.mddus.com

There are a number of other organisations you should consider joining:

The **British Medical Association** – the BMA is the trade union for doctors in Britain. Membership for students is reduced and brings with it many perks. You receive a monthly *Student BMJ*, access to online resources such as e-books and membership to the library services. If you are a student at a London Medical School or in London you can visit the BMA and benefit from the library amongst other services.

The BMA also has a national student committee consisting of representatives from each university. These positions are ideal for individuals who want to represent their university and have their voice heard, making a real difference to medical education and policy agendas on a national scale.

Further information can be found here: www.bma.org.uk

The **Royal Society for Medicine** is another organisation with a student branch. There are opportunities to join the student committee and represent your university again. Once again, this is a great opportunity to network with students from different universities and take advantage of the benefits on offer.

Further information can be found here: www.rsm.ac.uk

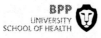

The **Royal College of Physicians** offers you insight into 30 specialties, clinical learning tools and discounts.

Further information can be found here: www.rcplondon.ac.uk / www.rcpe.ac.uk

The **Royal College of Surgeons** allows those with surgical interests to get involved with student events and courses. Medical students can join as affiliates.

Further information can be found here: www.rcseng.ac.uk / www.rcsed.ac.uk

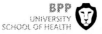

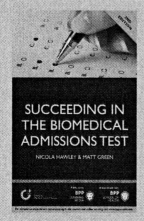
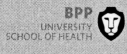

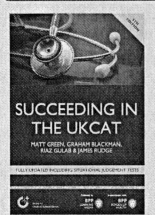
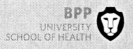

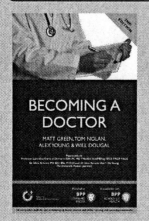

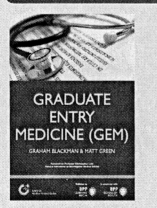
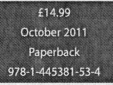
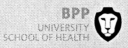

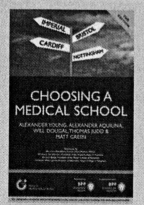
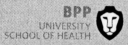

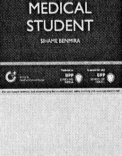